NEW

CALISTHENICS

FOR BEGINNERS

Table of Contents

INTRODUCTION…………………………….....4

CHAPTER ONE: WHAT IS CALISTHENICS?..9

CHAPTER TWO: THE ADVANTAGES AND DISADVANTAGES OF CALISTHENIC TRAINING……………………………………….17

CHAPTER THREE: MAJOR AREAS TO BE CONSIDERED FOR BEGINNER CALISTHENICS EXERCISE……………………28

CHAPTER FOUR: THE EQUIPMENTS USED IN CALISTHENICS…………………………………….42

CHAPTER FIVE: CALISTHENICS AND GOOD NUTRITION...66

CHAPTER SIX: REST AND RECOVERY.......102

CHAPTER SEVEN: PHYSICAL PREPARATION-1...116

CHAPTER EIGHT: PHYSICAL PREPARATION – 2...134

CHAPTER NINE: CALISTHENICS AND FLEXIBILITY EXERCISES...................146

CHAPTER TEN: ESSENTIAL EXERCISES IN CALISTHENICS...173

CHAPTER ELEVEN: ADDITIONAL EXERCISES IN CALISTHENICS.....................................183

CHAPTER TWELVE: APPLICATIONS OF CALISTHENICS TRAINING...............................194

CHAPTER THIRTEEN: AMPLIFYING YOUR BASIC WORKOUT......................................214

CHAPTER FOURTEEN: HEART RATE BOOSTING EXERCISES.................................223

CHAPTER FIFTEEN: RESTORATION AND FLEXIBILITY..232

CHAPTER SIXTEEN: MINDSET AND NURTURING HEALTHY HABITS...................260

CONCLUSION..278

INTRODUCTION

A great looking body, lots of strength and agility, and a positive mental outlook are the dream for most people. For those willing to put in 20 to 30 minutes a day at least three days a week performing a variety of calisthenics and bodyweight exercises, the dream can quickly become a reality!

Calisthenics (Cals) and Bodyweight training (BWT) has been around since the dawn of time – there were no gyms or fancy exercise equipment! Everyone has seen the movies with Roman gladiators, Greek warriors, and Nordic fighting men, and their physiques are all impressive! These images may come to us today from Hollywood, but the reality is also presented in countless museums across the globe in the shape of statues and paintings of real men and women.

There are also plenty of modern-day examples of excellent levels

of fitness achieved primarily through calisthenics and bodyweight training:

- Gymnasts

- Figure skaters

- Acrobats

- Martial arts experts

The human body is a fantastic machine, and it takes proper nutrition and maintenance in the form of functional movements to keep it functioning at an optimal level. Unfortunately, the availability of handy pre-prepared foods and labor-saving devices has caused people to lose sight of the best ways to keep healthy, and these habits are hard to break.

With just a little practice and determination, it is possible to reverse the effects of improper diet and inadequate activity at virtually any age and develop a strong, healthy, fit body that

looks good and leaves you feeling great.

In this book, you will be presented with an overview of how the body functions and the advantages of calisthenics and bodyweight training offer. You 're going to learn about:

• Discrepancies between Cals and BWT and other exercise styles

• How your body builds up and burns energy

• Suitable diet for feeding the body

• The effect that the mind has on exercise performance

• How to apply a wide variety of Cals and BWT exercises

• Main exercise routines and how to improve them

In other words, you will receive the information and motivation you need to start a Cals and BWT program and create your physical and mental outlook in the past. And without costly

facilities, gym memberships, or endless hours of exertion, this is all possible.

Happy Exercising!

CHAPTER ONE: WHAT IS CALISTHENICS?

To begin, it's worth taking a look at just what Calisthenics is, and what it's not, so we know whether certain exercises are included or not. Calisthenics history is a long one, and the word comes from the ancient Greek 'kallos,' meaning beauty, and 'sthenos,' meaning force. It can be called the art of using your own body weight and inertia qualities as a tool for improving your physique. For a little more of a detailed explanation, the concept of Calisthenics is as follows from Wikipedia:

Calisthenics is a form of physical training that consists of a variety of exercises, often rhythmic movements, usually without the use of equipment or device. With movements such as bending, running, spinning, twisting or punching, they are supposed to improve body strength and stability, using only

one's body weight for resistance. They are usually performed with stretches in concert. Calisthenics can support both physical and cardiovascular strength when practiced actively and with variety, in addition to improving psychomotor abilities such as balance, agility, and coordination.

Groups such as sports teams and military groups often carry out leading group calisthenics as a form of coordinated physical activity to improve group unity and discipline. Calisthenics is also popular in primary and secondary schools around the world, as a component of physical education.

In the ancient world, as part of their daily life and struggle to survive, the human race marched, raced, jumped, lunged, climbed, pushed, and pulled backward. Modern weights and machines found in commercial gyms are light years away from the kind of activity we as humans have been engaged in for

millennia, and that is why, at least in my opinion, Calisthenics is for us the most natural and comfortable type of exercise and movement to perform. Our relatives, the great apes, make use of this to develop tremendous power in the upper body, which can be seen with ease when watching Chimpanzees swing and climb trees and branches.

In time past, Calisthenics was used as the main source of the military's physical preparation, as it was easy to organize, easy to learn, and had the greatest transfer to the actual skills and movements needed by the soldiers. There was also something spiritual about being in tune with one's own body and being able to push it with no limitations or barriers across space. Technology also restricted what was possible, as it did not understand barbells, different weights, and the understanding of weighted movements. Still then, as the stories of Milo, Ares, and

Hercules attest, strength as a physical trait was respected and admired. For one thing, these famous and legendary figures were renowned, and that was their power and ability to use their muscles to exert force.

The elite gymnast is, without a doubt, the pinnacle of the calisthenics-type movement today. If there is another athlete who is bigger, more agile, more powerful, more versatile, or more mobile for pound, then I still have to hear of them. The interesting thing about gymnasts is that their strength can almost be seen as a by-product, as they usually train only for their event or discipline, and not for the potential to be strong. Even if this is the case, most gymnastics training takes place behind closed doors, and many practices upwards of thirty to forty hours a week, which is simply not possible for many people with the lives they lead. Moreover, a lot of gymnastics training is

traditionally done with an eye to ultimately advance and perfect the specific events and disciplines in which that particular gymnast will compete. For the person who just wants to be able to perform one-arm pull-ups or a front lever, most gymnastics training could be wasted on them, and even if it weren't, not everyone could devote or have the discipline to train like a gymnast.

Calisthenics has really seen a huge leap forward in recent years, in terms of its success and the campaigns being carried out. Anyone who reads this that is familiar with YouTube will have undoubtedly seen many amazing videos where ordinary people perform feats of inhuman strength and muscular control, using equipment no more advanced than a pull-up bar. This is the nature of what Calisthenics means, using the body to execute strength feats, which are seldom seen in other disciplines of

training. Another fascinating and admirable facet of modern Calisthenics is that most of the people involved in this type of training do not pay for a gym membership, do not have access to expensive equipment and do not have people telling them exactly what to do. In practice, they exercise in parks and basements, on pull-up bars and dip bars that they might have built themselves up to, yet they have more energy than most of the muscle heads that fill most of the modern world 's commercial gyms.

As a result, it is no surprise to see that Calisthenics also has a large place in parkour, or the tradition of free running. These men and women use grace and athleticism to perform powerful and daring feats where they run, jump, climb, push, and pull themselves over, under, and through road obstacles. Nearly all of these people are also well versed in the movements of Calisthenics and bodyweight strength, which makes this book

ideal for those who start free running or parkour. It is also that specialist workout competitions have risen in the last few years, where very strong men and women compete on a street workout course against each other. Some of the movements displayed here on the international gymnastics stage would not be out of place, such is the level of strength and athleticism shown.

Finally, Calisthenics is also used as a tool for other sports to build strength, as it helps to build a foundation that is not really available anywhere else. Even other forms of athletes, such as the Olympic Weightlifter, perform basic movements of Calisthenics to create a base level of strength before diverging and performing specific sporting examples. The name that most comes to mind is the one of Weightlifter Lu Xiaojun, the 77 kg World and Olympic champion. This is a man who can snatch 176 kg and clean and jerk 204 kg but is a daily staple of his training routine

for whom calisthenics and bodyweight exercise are. In many videos and pictures, he can be seen performing push-ups on the handstand, human flags, weighted dips, and other movements that would not look out of place in a street workout.

CHAPTER TWO: THE ADVANTAGES AND DISADVANTAGES OF CALISTHENIC TRAINING

Now that we've seen exactly what Calisthenics is, it's time to see what the advantages this training method offers. The first advantage is that everyone is somewhat used to exercising body weight as they have moved their own body weight through space since they were born. Therefore, the resistance is adapted to each individual; since it is his or her own bodyweight that is used as the resistance. I have often found that many people find it much easier to exercise with Calisthenics than they do when first handling dumbbells and barbells. This is good because it increases confidence and motivation. I can't tell you how many times I've told a customer that we're going to work with push-

ups, just to let them tell me they can't. Five minutes later, after I've shown them precisely how to perform a simple version, their faces light up as they remember they 're completely capable of performing Calisthenics, even if it's at a beginner level.

Second, compared with many other forms of exercise, injuring yourself performing Calisthenics isn't easy. This is for the simple reason that the strength or range of motion needed to be controlled is required to increase resistance using Calisthenics. Furthermore, this is not true of dumbbell and barbell exercises where excessive amounts of weight can be applied, even by complete novices, resulting in much higher injury risk. Moreover, many of the more difficult exercises can not simply be performed in Calisthenics; they have to be worked up to over a period of months and years before they can be regularly tried and trained. Compare this with weighted moves, where even a novice

will put 100 kg or 200lbs on a bar and attempt to squat with it.

The third advantage is that by increasing the leverage that can be brought to bear on the action, the complexity of the exercise can be made more demanding. The definition can be difficult to understand at first. In almost all other forms of exercise, more weight is simply added to the bar to increase the resistance, or a heavier weight is picked up and moved. But since we use Calisthenics we simply can not add more bodyweight. In order to increase the resistance, we must make it harder for the muscles to apply force. Think of carrying a heavy dumbbell or similar object in your hand to demonstrate this, with the weight falling by your side. The weight in question lies directly under the musculature in your shoulder, making it very easy to hold the position. Imagine now slowly shifting the weight to the side while keeping the elbow locked. This posture would become

increasingly difficult to maintain, and when the arm was horizontal, the movement would become the most difficult to maintain. At this level, the ability of the shoulder muscles to exert pressure on the weight is reduced, resulting in the need for more pressure to maintain the position. It makes the muscle stronger over time as there has been little improvement in the actual weight lifted. This idea of manipulating an exercise's leverage is extensively used in this book, particularly for the more challenging movements. As you progress through the book, you'll notice that exercises like the front lever, back lever, pseudo planche push-up, and many others all rely on this leverage manipulation method to increase the exercise 's difficulty.

The fourth advantage is that the power generated from Calisthenics can be applied to a wide range of sports and athletic activities. There are many hypotheses that try to explain why this

is so, and they can all be equally valid. My own personal opinion is that almost all movements in Calisthenics, and particularly the more advanced ones, teach the body how to act as a complete unit. If we use the planche as an example, this exercise requires that all the muscles in the body act as one, with the maximum tension needed for the action to be carried out. This is especially useful because for some people, especially the young and undertrained, weighted movements and barbell and dumbbell moves are not suitable. The use of Calisthenics helps anyone to build a solid basis of strength from which to proceed.

Calisthenics' fifth advantage is that it makes good use of the isometric exercises. Isometric exercises are the ones where the muscles are under tension but are not getting shorter or longer. It would be a real-world example of an isometric contraction to push against a locked door or solid wall. This is unlike intense

contractions, where under tension, the muscles get shorter or eccentric contractions, where under stress, the muscles get longer. Isometric exercises are different from normal exercises because they do not count reps; instead, the exercises are held for a set amount of time. There is no clear way to replicate weight-related isometric calisthenics exercises, and the type of force that can be generated with these locked, static positions is special. An example is the half-lever, which is seen next.

DISASVANTAGES OF CALISTHENICS

Although there are many benefits to performing Calisthenics, there are also a few drawbacks, and it is worth considering these before we make progress.

The first downside is that it can be difficult to build enormous

strength in the lower body using just your own bodyweight as the resistance because no weights are used. The lower body includes the largest and most powerful muscles in the body, like the quadriceps and glutes. This means they must contract a lot of resistance to obtain any gains in strength. The unfortunate fact is that there are not a large number of calisthenics exercises that we can use to provide sufficient resistance to create enormous force. Bodyweight squats, single-legged squats, lungs, and hamstring curls are some of the exercises we'll look at later in the book, and although they build up enormous amounts of energy, I personally found that my legs were far behind the rest of my body when I started training with Olympic Weightlifting and front and back squats. This is, of course, only a concern if lower body strength is important to you or the specific ability to squat large loads. If this is not the case, then don't worry.

The second drawback is that it is difficult to design exercises that incorporate decreased leverage principles because of the way the lower body is built. There are many exercises in the upper body that rely on this principle to maximize strength gains, such as the planche, the front and back lever, and many others. There's no way around this reality, which is why you see the person on almost every calisthenics video either doesn't look like he trains legs, or doesn't do any lower body exercises. In my view, this is a shame because training the lower body will aid immensely in building muscle and developing strength in the rest of the body.

The third downside is that because weight can not be applied to raise resistance, except in the case of weighted pull-ups, etc., then we will rely on the method of reducing the amount of leverage to make the movement easier. Although this is an incredibly successful way of making an exercise more difficult, it

is not the same as rising the load on a barbell every few weeks by a couple of kilograms or pounds. For example, if we were doing the bench press, we could be very precise in keeping track of exactly how much weight we were lifting and how much each week or month it was through. We can not do that with Calisthenics. Of course, we can keep track of how many repetitions we have made, or how much our range of motion has improved, and how long we have kept those positions, but in terms of tracking progress, calisthenics training is much less precise.

Some people challenge the fourth downside but still remains a common belief, which is that performing Calisthenics can not create loads of muscle. I don't believe that is true, simply because of the presence of some of the people I've seen performing movements in Calisthenics. A quick perusal on YouTube will

show there are some seriously built guys doing nothing apart from exercise in body weight. It is true that there is actually a limit to the size of the muscle that can be provided to you by Calisthenics, but if you want bodybuilder size then it will make sense for you to only do bodybuild. If you want extreme, superhuman strength, decent size, and great tone of the muscle, then Calisthenics is the way ahead.

CHAPTER THREE: MAJOR AREAS TO BE CONSIDERED FOR BEGINNER CALISTHENICS EXERCISE

Because Calisthenics is a particular type of training and exercise, it has its own unique advantages and disadvantages, and I would like to take some time to go over these here. These aspects are due to the way calisthenics exercises use the body's muscles, as well as the equipment that is being used, or lack thereof. This implies that it is possible to use Calisthenics to improve forms of strength and endurance that can not be developed naturally or by other techniques.

HAND STRENGTH

The first peculiar feature of Calisthenics is that almost every single movement we look at involves the hands. Pushing,

pulling, and core exercises all use the hands to a large extent, and because Calisthenics stresses complete control and the strength of the whole body, supports such as belts and hooks are not used at all. It compares with bodybuilding and other weighted types of exercise, where belts are used to help people stay on pull-up bars, and hooks are used to help support the barbell as it rises to death. You'll have no doubt seen this being done in gyms, by almost everybody trying to get solid. The use of hooks and braces is part and parcel of the sport for the bodybuilder; they tend to hit other muscles, so they don't want the hands, so forearms to tire until the main muscle on which they operate gets tired. Furthermore, we, as practitioners of Calisthenics want the hands and forearms to be as solid as physically possible, and by extension, the grip. This makes complete sense when you're giving it a thought for a moment. You may have the strongest back in the world, but it is useless if your hands and forearms are

not powerful enough to pass the power and make use of it. I am such a believer in the strength of my hand that I have written a whole book on the subject, called GRIP.

You use your hands in Calisthenics for many things; hold onto the floor and control your body weight, grab a pull-up bar and hang from objects, and move from one position to another using sheer energy rather than momentum. All these activities depend on the strength of hand and finger, and if you don't have that, you probably won't be able to do any of the more advanced calisthenics movements. Of course, there are different hand and finger strength exercises that can be used to directly target the muscles that are used for gripping, but much of the strength needed can and will be obtained by simply performing the basic exercises I've set out in the exercise section.

THE CORE

The heart is a part of the body that, over the years, has seen its fair share of fad exercises and devices, and I think we can all say confidently that most of them are absolute crap. Contrary to popular belief, or what the media can tell you, doing thousands of sit-ups or crunches won't build a strong heart. Doing crunches and sit-ups won't burn any fat off your midsection either. In terms of what it needs to get better, the core musculature is no different from any other muscle fiber. To get stronger, a muscle needs to contract against a resistance, and the resistance needs to increase over time in order for that strength to grow. Take note of that sentence: it is not the sum of repetitions that must increase; it is the resistance that must increase. This means that no matter how many sit-ups you do if

you don't increase the resistance, your body won't get stronger.

In traditional exercise, the core is seen simply as a part of the body to be improved aesthetically. The abs are worked on, diet is strictly adhered to, and everybody needs a six-pack. However, the heart plays a vital role in Calisthenics, and is not merely relegated to the back seat. Many exercises that can be called calisthenic require that the core keep the body's midline completely steady. If we do an exercise like the front lever, we can see that although it is hugely reliant on the pulling strength of the upper body, the core also has to keep the whole body straight and also hold the weight of the legs. This means that a core built using calisthenics exercises will be among the most powerful you'll ever encounter.

Since we need to increase resistance to increase strength, this means we have to do a lot of the more conventional core

exercises to get rid of. This doesn't mean that this book doesn't contain easier or simpler core movements, it does, but it just doesn't mean that those alone can't be relied on to build the core strength level we need if we want to progress to a decent standard.

The more advanced core exercises, many of which you may not have seen before, such as the half lever, are very common in gymnastics circles and develop such enormous core strength that, once mastered, can make other core exercises look like child's play. Be in no doubt that if you are able to execute some of the more complex moves, you can fairly claim to have one of the strongest cores around.

THE SCAPULA

Forget big shoulders and wide backs; a person's ability to balance and control his / her scapula is the real home of upper body strength. The scapulas, more generally referred to as the shoulder blades, is the point at which the arms' bones and muscles join the shoulder, and the scapula is the point at which they merge. Essentially, the scapula is capable of four movements, which are acceleration, fall, protraction, and retraction. When you shrug your shoulders up or move your shoulders to your ears, elevation happens. Depression happens when you cause your shoulders to fall into the bottom. Retraction occurs as you draw your head back and puff your arms, and when you round the back and move your spine and shoulder blades apart, protraction happens.

If the scapula can be rendered as powerful as possible, then any strength you build in the rest of the upper body can be

transferred much more effectively. Of all the body parts involved in the movements of Calisthenics, particularly the advanced ones, the scapula is probably the most important but least understood. The scapula houses the musculature of the rotator cuff, described by Wikipedia as following;

The rotator cuff muscles are essential for shoulder movements and for preserving the stability of the shoulder joint. Such muscles come from the scapula and attach to the humerus' back, forming a band at the joint of the shoulder. We keep the humerus head within the scapula's small and shallow glenoid fossa. Analogously the glenohumeral joint was described as a golf ball sitting on a golf tee.

The rotator cuff muscles also perform multiple functions, including abduction, internal rotation, and external shoulder rotation, while stabilizing the glenohumeral joint and regulating

humeral head translation. Infraspinatus and subscapularis have significant roles in the abduction of the shoulder of the scapular plane, producing forces two to three times greater than the force produced by the muscle of the supraspinate. However, because of its moment arm, the supraspinatus is more effective for general shoulder abduction. The anterior portion of the tendon supraspinatus is subjected to significantly higher load and stress and plays its main functional role.

If you're not physiologically inclined, the above description may seem like a load of nonsense, but the first sentence is all we need to take away from it. The rotator cuff muscles are essential for shoulder movements and for preserving the stability of the shoulder joint.

Your success in many of the most difficult movements of Calisthenics relies on the ability of your rotator cuff muscles to

stabilize the shoulder joint, allowing the other muscle groups to do the actual work. It refers to pull-ups, frames, front levers, one-arm chin-ups, and many other movements involving extreme strength. In the book's mobility section, I will describe some exercises that are important for shoulder health that should be done by everyone, irrespective of your starting strength level.

STRAIGHT-ARM STRENGTH

Calisthenics, and much of the gymnastics by extension, places heavy emphasis on a phenomenon known as straight-arm power. Even if you don't know this definition, you'll have no doubt seen it being used. It is used by gymnasts on television when performing movements on the still hoops, as in the iron cross and crucifix, or when demonstrating their abilities on the planche.

The straight-arm strength is exactly what it sounds like; the energy with a locked elbow was applied. This puts enormous strain on the arm and its connective tissues, including the biceps and the tendon of the biceps, as well as the hands and wrists. Movements such as the planche, which we will discuss in detail later on the book, use straight-arm power without which it would be difficult or impossible to execute. This feat is also the reason that many gymnasts and calisthenics practitioners have very large biceps, although they do not do any kind of typical biceps curl exercises. The strain on the elongated muscle makes it a dramatic amount to increase in size and strength, and also allows for many of the more advanced calisthenics exercises.

The excellent side-effect of pulling with a straight arm is that it makes the back extremely strong. If the arm is held straight, then, the back muscles have to work incredibly hard to exert

some force on the floor. Obviously, this increases strength in a way that is not replicable in any other form. This is also why calisthenics and gymnastics practitioners have outstanding back musculature. There are a number of exercises in this book which depend on straight-arm power. The planche, front lever, back lever, and human flag are just some of the moves that will expose you to this unique and novel aspect of Calisthenics.

TRAINING THE NERVOUS SYSTEM

Another very unique aspect of Calisthenics is that of the nervous system being trained, which is only really experienced when doing extremely intense workouts. Instead of being mentioned, this is better experienced, but is actually the body being taxed and strained so much that you feel as though it has worked more than your muscles have.

This facet of Calisthenics is most practiced when dealing with movements involving lots of groups of muscles at the same time or requiring lots and lots of muscle tension to be maintained for extended periods. Sources of this are the planche, front, back, and half levers, and very complicated moves like the pull-up of one arm. You should find that you can not simply repeat these exercises indefinitely, as the body becomes tired and drained after a short time. This is natural and is just an indication that the exercise does its job.

This can also be seen in strongman training and weightlifting and powerlifting. Imagine going in for a deadlift of 1 rep max. An exercise like this needs so much energy to be generated that you simply cannot continue to do it again and again. You may be able to go for a few reps, but your body will become exhausted after that. This is exactly the same thing that happens with the

motions of high-level Calisthenics but simply by using exercises

of body weight.

CHAPTER FOUR: THE EQUIPMENTS USED IN CALISTHENICS

The beauty of using an exercise method such as Calisthenics is

that there is hardly any equipment required for you to do the

workouts. All you need to have an extremely effective calisthenics workout can often be found at any playground or play park. There you can find pull-up bars, dip bars, vertical bars, monkey bars, and several other pieces of equipment as long as it is considered safe for you to practice there. There are also specialist fitness areas in several countries with several different styles of bar configurations, including various heights and thicknesses. Those are not that popular though, so you don't have to worry if you don't live near one of these places.

That's not to suggest you should only use something to execute moves and movements on. Many books I've seen dealing with bodyweight exercise suggest the comprehensive use of household items during your workouts. For a number of reasons, that is a very bad idea. Number one is that the vast majority of household objects are not designed for you to do pull-ups, dips, and other

exercises on them, depending on your own weight. When they crash or break while using them, you 're going to get hurt.

Calisthenics also has the added advantage of getting hold of the equipment and appliances you need would be really easy. The material from which the equipment is produced is most often inexpensive, readily available, and is not difficult to build. This contrasts sharply with friction plates, treadmills, cross trainers, rowing machines, weight plates, and Olympic bars, etc., which can be very expensive to buy and maintain. You will find that no need to retain pull-up and dip bars!

Over the next few parts, we will look at the various types of equipment that can be used to conduct calisthenics training on, where to find it, and how important each piece is to your success.

LOCATION FOR TRAINING

The first thing to decide when you start training your Calisthenics is where to train. This is a big decision because the most important thing is that you enjoy your preparation, because if you don't find a suitable position, then you are much more likely to give up. There are numerous locations that can be appropriate, and I'm going to run through a few of those here.

First, for calisthenics preparation, commercial gyms and fitness clubs can be fantastic, and virtually anyone reading this book can live relatively close to one of these facilities. The advantages are that they usually have plenty of equipment; they 're indoors, so the training schedule won't be disrupted by the environment, and the prices are low. The downside is that you'll pay for a lot of services (such as swimming pools, etc.) that you may not get a lot of use from. Also, the type of equipment they do have would

not be absolutely conducive to Calisthenics. Cross Fit gyms are one form of exercises that is really good for the Calisthenics. Whatever your opinion, and I have many on Cross Fit, it can not be denied that they have some very good facilities with equipment that is pretty much perfect for those interested in doing Calisthenics.

Second, playgrounds and play parks are another viable choices for those who want to practice using Calisthenics but don't want to enter a gym or spend any money on equipment. These days, most playgrounds have different pull-up bars, dip bars, monkey bars, tables, ropes, etc., which can be much, much easier to use than a commercial gymnasium. The downsides are that almost all playgrounds and parks are outdoors, and if you're hoping to use such a location for your training, you'll have to deal with the environment. If you have a warm and dry place, then that's not a

problem, but it's still a problem to consider. The other is for defense. Playgrounds are often built for children, and problems with adults working out in close proximity to children can arise. It would be better to consult with the local authority, in this case, to see if it will be appropriate for you to train there. Alternatively, you could just wait until the kids went home, and that wouldn't be a problem then.

The third choice is to use an area explicitly designed as a training area for bodyweight and Calisthenics. If you live in the U.S. or Eastern Europe or Russia, they are becoming increasingly common, especially within the city, where they can normally be found next to or joined to basketball courts. These are less common in England but are becoming increasingly accessible as a result of initiatives to activate young people. Such types of workout areas usually have a multitude of different height and

bar thickness pull-up bars, dip bars, parallels, etc. The other great thing in these places is that there will be other people there who want to learn as you do and having learning buddies and groups is one of the best ways to improve.

The last place you can train is within your house. This will require buying or making some equipment yourself, as it is unlikely that you will have a ready-made calisthenics gym at the house you buy or move into. However, this doesn't mean you need to spend a lot because most of the equipment required for calisthenics training is very inexpensive and easy to get. During the next segment, we will look at some of the pieces of equipment used for calisthenics and bodyweight training, what it should have, where it can be found, and alternatives to the products purchased.

THE PULL-UP BAR

While equipment is not really required for Calisthenics, performing all of the pulling exercises without anything to pull on is very difficult, probably impossible. A pull-up bar is the perfect piece of equipment for that. Not only can a pull-up bar be used for all pulling exercises, but it can also be used for most core exercises, and even some of the pushing exercises. That may make it the most cost-effective piece of exercise equipment ever made. Both gyms are expected to have these, and if they don't, don't enter or change gyms. If they don't have the most basic piece of equipment for Calisthenics then I am afraid to think what else they don't have. If you're fortunate, they'll have a bar not close to the wall, allowing you to work on muscle-ups in a timely manner. If you are not a member of a gym, on the other hand, and have no intention of ever joining one, then there are a

range of choices for you.

You can buy one pull-up bar first. When you follow this path, then it will definitely be one of the best choices you can make on your physical fitness journey. There are different styles of pull-up bars, ranging from those that bolt to walls, to those that fit into door frames and even standing alone. You will be able to find one that is relatively easily tailored to your budget and living situation. I use a PowerBar * at home, which I have been in dutiful usage for a few years now. It never let me down and was very inexpensive, and it tends to suit a wide range of door frames.

Whether you can't afford a pull-up panel, or you can install one nowhere, then there are a variety of alternatives. One is to use any object that's above your head that you can grab. This might include stairs below in a basement or cellar, a balcony, or even a

branch of a tree. As long as the item in question can bear your weight safely, then I see no reason why pulling exercises on can't be used.

DIP BARS

Dip bars are another common piece of equipment found not only in commercial gymnasiums but also in play parks and training areas outside. They are usually used for triceps dips as the name implies, but can also be used for all sorts of exercises, like front and back levers, muscle-ups, and handstand and planche function. The dip bars found in commercial gyms are often attached to a larger piece of equipment, such as pull-up bars and leg raise stations, so these may not be good for a pure calisthenics workout at times, but can still be used effectively. The dip bars are also much longer in play parks, which means

that two or three people can exercise at the same time, or you can ride along with them, turn around, do handstands, planks, etc., and really get a good workout. Dip bars can come in several different variations, with different bar thicknesses, widths, and heights, as with pull-up bars. It's rare to find stand-alone units you can buy, but if you're looking over the internet, you might find some.

Since I've got the space in my home, I've built a set of dip bars in my back garden, and if you have space and the spare time, I strongly encourage you to do that as well (as long as the wife/husband/partner/parents of course allow). Building your own means you can customize the width for your own body shape and type, you can make the bar as thick or as thin as you like. If you're interested in doing this, then a prompt Google search will pull up loads of tutorials on how to do this.

PARALLETS

In some ways, parallets are similar to dip bars, in that they consist of two bars that are a set distance apart, and facing the same. The difference is that parallets are typically compact and slightly lower to the ground. If you've ever seen push-up bars, parallets are just bigger models. Parallets can be used to drive movements like push-ups, handstands, planche work, etc. The advantage is that you can broaden and narrow the grip as they are separate units to match your unique type of body. Even they can be carried almost anywhere because they are so small and portable. This is ideal if you travel a lot, or are away on business, or simply don't have much room to build a training area in your home.

Parallets come in different types, but there are a variety of things

you should look for when you buy them:

- The first is they have to be robust. This is for motives that are clear. If you're in a handstand, you don't want the tool you 're using to malfunction because you're most likely going to hurt yourself and others.

- The second is they need a bar width that's comfortable to hold onto. Using parallets that have a diameter of a few inches is not good, and although that would do wonders for your grip strength, it will make it much harder to control handstands and boards and other exercises. There are a number of places you can buy online parallets, so it's best to just have a look around and see what you can find.

- As I did, the third option is to make your own. It is really straightforward, and a lot of money can be saved. There's a lot of instructional videos and guides out there that will teach

you how to make fitness equipment on the internet, like parallets. Doing a fast search will produce a decent number of results, but on my own parallels the basic structure can be seen, an image of which is shown next.

I took, as you can see, a single piece of thick dowel, about 30 mm in diameter, and cut it halfway. Then I stacked up tiny wooden squares until I had four towers about 10 to 12 inches high. These were then screwed together, and the dowel ends fastened to the four towers. Clearly, they look really handmade, but I've had these for about five years now, and once they didn't disappoint me.

It is important to make sure that you place the correct width apart when using parallets. That's going to be special to every individual, but the easiest way is to put them apart, so they're shoulder width. This ensures that your hands should be placed

directly below your shoulders as you do planks, handstands, half levers, etc. This will make supporting yourself much easier because your arms will behave like vertical columns that support the rest of your body weight. You can either look at yourself in a mirror to see the width of your shoulder, or you can get a training partner to help. If you can't do that, your shoulder width would usually be the same as the distance from your fingertip to your elbow. Simply position your comparisons according to this equation, and you'll be well off.

CHOOSING THE APPROPRIATE OUTFIT

The type of clothing that you wear isn't really that important, but there are a couple of things to remember. First, whatever you have chosen to wear to exercise and train in will give your body full freedom of movement, without any limitations on the joints.

The way that strength is built in Calisthenics is by using the full range of motion in every workout, and if that is hindered by the clothes you 're wearing, then you're going to get off to a bad start. My favorite apparel is usually loose-fitting shorts and a t-shirt or jacket, or if I'm training somewhere that allows me to go shirtless, then I'm going to train without a shirt. Training without a shirt has many benefits, such as greater freedom of movement, less resistance to joint movement, and also allowing the body to better control its temperature. No-shirt training often helps you to track the movements more closely and to see what the body is doing at all times. This is invaluable if you have a training partner because they would be able to tell you when you're going wrong and where you're doing it right, particularly when practicing and feeling the correct body position for exercises like the back lever etc.

Secondly, do not think you need to spend a great deal of money on fitness clothes. You will be doing muscle-ups and other movements soon, where the clothes material will come into contact with the bars and other surfaces, and that is one of the best ways to ruin a good t-shirt. Moreover, contrary to what the big sports brands might tell you, their clothing won't turn you into a king of Calisthenics overnight, so do yourself a favor and save some money.

CHALK

Many of the exercises in this book require a very strong and stable grip, particularly those requiring heavy use of the hands and the upper body. For example, the false grip, which is a technique used on the pull-up bar for muscle-ups, depends on the hands not shifting from a set position, or it will not be

possible to compete effectively with the motion. To that end, making sure that your grip is not slipping due to sweat from your hands or a slippery surface on the piece of equipment is of great importance. It is here that chalk comes in. Chalk effectively dries out the hands and provides a more abrasive and stickier surface for operating with the grip. There are two main chalk types, and we're going to discuss them both here.

The first is the typical powdered chalk that gymnasts, weightlifters, and climbers may have used to help you see. This usually comes in large square blocks, which are then broken down and placed in some sort of container. There are many downsides to this, including excess chalk on the floor and on the appliance, chalk dust in the air that can be breathed in and make its way into the eyes, and the task of re-applying the chalk after a short time.

The second type is liquid chalk, usually occurring in a small bottle. Liquid chalk is the same compound as regular powdered chalk, except for adding a liquid that evaporates from the skin once it is applied. It leaves a thin layer of chalk on the palm surface of the hand, which makes it much easier to grip pull-up bars and parallets. Liquid chalk also doesn't have to be re-applied as often as powdered chalk, doesn't get into the air or the lungs or eyes, and can also be applied to wrists and other areas of the body that can't be applied.

If you are a member of a gym, then it's worth testing whether they allow the use of chalk on pull-up bars and other equipment. I 'd consider changing gyms if they don't because they obviously care more about the condition of their floors or bars than about the strength and fitness goals.

FOAM ROLLER

While a foam roller isn't really vital, it may be handy for mobility drills and muscle and tissue maintenance. Simply put, Self Myofascial Release, or more simply, Foam Rolling, uses a foam roller. Foam rolling is the act of putting pressure on and rolling over a muscle or muscle group using the body's own weight as the force. This can help align muscle fibers, release muscle fascia, and also remove any sore parts, scar tissue, and knots in the muscle fiber.

Foam rollers can be purchased from many sources, and some of these should be in possession of most good commercial gyms. These generally come in different densities, with the lighter rollers ideal for beginners and the heavier ones perfect for those who have been rolling foam for a while. If especially for your training, you don't want to buy a foam roller, then you can use

many household objects to achieve much the same result. It can be used to foam roll tennis balls, cardboard tubes, plumbing pipes, and many other things.

TRAINING PARTNER

A Training Partner is the last piece of optional equipment. You will either have people lining up to train alongside you, or those who make every excuse under the sun not to exercise, depending on your social circle and the sort of individuals who are your friends. If you can find someone who will be able to take part in a regular training partner, you will be lucky. A training partner can really make the difference, especially when it comes to pushing you through the plateaus and hitting new highs. You will often find that training with someone else will help to create a healthy dose of rivalry and competition, which is always good

for progress and improvement. We will also be able to watch,

you do the exercises and tell you where you're wrong, and when

you're doing the right things.

CHAPTER FIVE: CALISTHENICS AND GOOD NUTRITION

Now that you understand what Calisthenics is and what kind of strength it will give you, it's time to look at a very important part of all physical training that is nutrition, rest, and recovery. Many people make the training mistake very hard, but then don't eat properly, rest enough, or sleep enough, and then fail to recover and get stronger afterward. This next part of the book aims to provide you with all the details you need regarding the right diet, the right amount of rest time, and the right amount and type of sleep.

Nutrition is actually a simple idea, but sadly, the basic principles are not being taken into account by many people. Processed, processed, and fast food has become the standard, and through modern ways of managing, the balanced quality of whole food has been lost to a great extent. Since fiber and many of the essential minerals have been stripped away from the foods we consume, this has undermined the function of the human body. Convenience has a lot of people overloading carbohydrates and fats, resulting in an ever-increasing line of the waist and a slow look.

If you are serious about building real power and strength, then you need to get your diet right. If you also want your body fat to decrease and get ripped, then diet becomes more important. Since there's so much money to make these days, a new diet is invented nearly every day. This fact means the garbage is present

in the vast majority of diets and food plans. Most nutritionists and dietitians complicate things far too much, thinking that if they do, you will become forever dependent on their advice and knowledge. Complicating things in my experience just causes problems, while keeping things simple means making the plan easier to follow and more effective.

Read every fitness magazine, and see a number of different rules and regulations to eat a good diet. For the first week, some will claim to monitor calories, some will suggest not to eat sugar, and some will have traffic light systems for various foods. All those diets and eating strategies are, in my opinion, more hassle than they are worth. Building substantial strength in Calisthenics needs a lot of physical preparation, so we don't want to waste time trying to eat a really complicated way. In this next section, I have listed a number of diet and nutritional rules which are easy

to follow and should make perfect sense.

EAT MORE OF NATURAL FOODS

Real food is the minimally processed food, which either runs, swims, flies, or grows. All sources of natural food are meat, fish, poultry, eggs, nuts, fruit, and vegetables. That is a very straightforward law. The more natural food you eat, the better, as it will provide more and more nutrients and will be better suited to the digestive system in your body. Whether you eat organic foods or not is up to you. There's plenty of evidence to show you organic food is no better than non-organic food, but that doesn't make any sense to me. I don't eat strictly organic food, but if you are worried about pesticides and herbicides that contaminate your food, it would be a good idea to think about it.

A mix of nutrients is best with respect to what food to eat. It means your protein's meat, fish, eggs and dairy, plenty of fruits and vegetables for your carbs, and your milk, olive oil, and nuts, and seed fat. Contrary to popular belief, eating an all-natural diet isn't more expensive than eating junk food, and even if it was, that's not yet a reason to eat junk food. It can also be known as the diet with a single ingredient. If you eat only natural food, then all the food you eat will consist of one ingredient. In this respect, it is the easiest diet ever invented to adopt. Simply hold it in your hand when selecting food, and ask yourself if it has one ingredient or not. If it does, eat it; if it does not eat it, then eat it not. Quite straightforward.

EAT BIG TO GAIN BIG MUSCLES

Most of you would like to read this to put on muscle mass, either

for esthetic purposes or to make exercises of strength more manageable. You simply have to take in more calories and bring on the body than you consume, but these calories must be of good quality. Sometimes this was rendered as "eat big to get tall." If you're training for strength, then you'll certainly feel the need to eat more, so don't feel bad about that. Strength training is extremely taxing on the body, and you will need to consume food and nutrients in abundance so that the body will have the resources to fix itself. We've been used to learning about regular intake of calories for adults, whether you live in a western world or not, and in my opinion, these have skewed almost everyone's understanding of what constitutes a healthy diet.

If you're practicing for strength, then you'll need to eat a lot more than prescribed by doctors and other health professionals. Read every interview with the toughest men on the planet right

now as an extreme example; men like Brian Shaw, Benedikt Magnusson, and others, and you will often hear them say they eat nearly 10,000 calories a day! This is because you have to eat when you're training for strength, and you need to eat a lot.

One drawback to eating lots of food, even if it's the natural food of very good quality, is that there's a chance that you'll put on body fat. To some extent, this is inevitable, which is why bodybuilders must go through a bulking and dieting process, where they will eat and put on muscle in the first step, and then and their calories and body fat. Don't think about this too much, because once you've reached a point where you've put on the muscle mass you want, you will reduce the amount of food you consume and drop body fat.

INCREASE YOUR PROTEIN CONSUMPTION

Protein is probably the most essential of all the macronutrients

(the others being carbohydrates and fats) when it comes to strength training. That is because protein is the element responsible for muscle development and maintenance. Eating enough protein-containing food will help you retain the muscle you already have, which is vital for the obvious reasons. Protein can be found in meat such as beef, pork and lamb, fish, eggs, milk, cheese and other dairy products, and legumes, nuts, and seeds of all kinds. If you eat a relatively varied diet, you should have no problem getting enough protein into your body, especially if you're not a vegetarian.

If you are a vegetarian, then you can still build muscle and strength, as will be shown by the example of most vegetarian animals around the world. The only problem that some vegetarians have is that if you eat a purely vegetarian one, there may be some amino acids missing from your diet because animal

protein has a complete amino acid profile. This can be rectified with various supplements, and if you are a vegetarian, it is worth looking into.

This can and does vary based on a variety of variables, including your ethnicity, history of training, body size, the strength of training, and many other factors, as to the amount of protein you'll need. For every pound of lean body weight, a rough guide is to take one gram of protein, or two grams of protein for every kilogram of body weight. For instance, if you weigh 80 kilograms or 160 pounds, then 160 grams of protein a day is a target you should aim for. Do not think too much about this, because most people take in enough protein per day to stop counting the number of grams you eat. If you're just trying to eat some protein at each meal, you won't have trouble getting enough in your body.

REDUCE YOUR INTAKE OF CARBOHYDRATES

There's one form of food available nowadays more readily than ever before, which causes more health issues than any other, and this food is processed carbohydrate. Refined carbohydrates contain white flour, white bread, pasta, white rice, sugar and pastry and for a variety of reasons, they are bad for you:

First, at four calories per gram, they have a fairly high energy density. It isn't as big as sugar, at nine calories per gram, but people don't eat near the amount of sugar anywhere as they do carbs, which is the main reason so many people have weight issues. They steer clear of sugar, eat low-fat yogurt, milk, cheese, etc., but do not dream about eating bread loaves, pasta, rice, potatoes, and other starchy carbohydrates of any kind.

Second, consuming tons of carbohydrates can and will spike blood sugar, which can then lead to increased fat retention, blunted insulin response, and other side effects that are not beneficial for us, particularly those who are training for strength and efficiency.

Thirdly, they 're intolerant to yeast and gluten to some degree for many people, at least in the western world. Especially in bread and most types of flour, yeast and gluten are found, which is often the cause of the bloated feeling you get. This is because of the proteins in the gluten that cause inflammation in the intestine, which is not a desirable situation for us as we should be busy recovering from a strength workout, not trying to fight inflammation. If you can study the Paleolithic diet or the Caveman diet, it will tell you why eating wheat, or grains, in general, isn't such a good idea for humans.

Finally, if you are looking to get ripped or reduce your body fat, it's the best thing you can do to reduce your intake of refined carbohydrates. Refined carbohydrates are very energy-dense, and eating a lot of them will make a substantial contribution to your body fat intake.

UNDERSTANDING WHAT THE BODY NEEDS

The phrase 'a well-balanced diet' has been heard by many, but what does that actually mean? The body requires food from a wide variety of sources to provide the routine safe functioning requirements such as:

- Duck, fowl, lean meat, and nut proteins
- Fruits and vegetables
- Whole grain

- Mackerel

- Healthy fats and oils

- Restricted amounts of processed feed, potatoes, white rice (carbohydrates!)

- Only small amounts of other products, such as salt, sugar, and processed food.

Dieting is generally a bad idea since most people are so wrong about it. If someone wants to go on a diet, the direction appears to be a dramatic transition, resulting in a considerable amount of stress on the body that they respond to with drastic steps. It ensures that in case the 'famine' lasts a while, the metabolism must slow down to save the available resources. So as you eat less and fewer calories, the body uses less and less of these for essential functions.

Even carbohydrate cutting causes problems because these complex chains perform other functions besides 'making you fat.' It takes carbohydrates for:

- Cellular development and how it operates

- Blood sugar levels controlled

- Helps regulate blood pressure and control cholesterol levels

- Provision of probiotic nutrients which promote proper digestion

- To absorb calcium

- CNS- and brain fuel

Particularly when you decide to start an exercise routine, you should take a close look at what you use to fuel your body. Endurance athletes 'flash carbs'-in other words, eat vast quantities of carbohydrates during athletic activity for the glucose they can supply. However, unlike these athletes, most

people are eating more than enough carbohydrates to meet their workout needs. Some carbs like processed sugar and wheat products should be avoided or limited, but there are a lot of other healthy carbohydrate sources. The main factor is not necessarily the amount but the source of the carbohydrates.

Eating an exceptionally high protein diet can be harmful to a variety of reasons as well. Because burning body fat and the protein available causes a buildup of ketones (the product of burning these fuel sources), this can lead to an imbalance in the body's chemistry resulting in acidosis, unpleasant bad breath, and body odor and even a coma. A diet program is based on this principle but must be carefully monitored. Muscle tissue consists of protein so that the body can potentially start consuming its own tissues for fuel when there is not enough protein available to sustain the muscle. Limiting certain types of foods can lead to

constipation and illness due to inadequate vitamins.

Rather than looking at a diet as the need to cut out all foods, it should be looked at as a balanced strategy to include the correct proportions of all the nutrients the body needs. By adding fuel of higher quality, your body will work better, and you will feel better, too.

PICK A HEALTHY DIET

There are several different sources explaining the 'ideal' diet, but it is possible to break down the basic guidelines as follows:

1. Whole grains (cereal, bread, pasta, and rice) and other carbohydrates like barley, cornmeal, beans, flax, and quinoa – 6 – 11 servings a day

2. Clean, organic fruits and vegetables – 5 – 9 servings a day
    (raw is the best option for many of these)

3. Dairy items include milk, cheese, and yogurt – 2 to 4
    servings a day

4. Meat, fowl, lean meat, eggs, nuts, and beans protein – 2
    – 3 servings a day

5. Healthy fats and oils-monounsaturated fats like corn,
    sunflower, peanut and sesame oil and avocados, olives
    and a range of nuts like peanuts, hazelnuts, almonds,
    pecans, cashews, and macadamia nuts

6. Very limited quantities of potatoes, white rice, and
    refined, processed grains (this is what most people see as
    carbohydrates, and they should be eliminated!)

7. Minimum amounts of other products, including salt,
    sugar, processed foods, and alcohol.

8. Another important issue for people who need to limit their intake of food to reduce calories is the regulation of portions. What you see on most plates is considerably more than just a suitable part! In some cases, one meal may contain more calories than a whole day's needs!

- One serving is 3 oz of meat. -- Around the size of a soap bar or a checkbook.

- Cooked pasta is the size of a fist (1/2 cup).

- A CD case should be about the size of the toast, waffles or pancakes

- 4 Dice shaped cheese cubes make up one serving

- Fresh vegetables and fruit (about 1 cup) should have the size of a baseball or tennis ball

Measuring food is the easiest way of serving sufficient portion sizes. However, for most people, that is quite problematic, so

one way to get around is to measure basic portions with water and pour it into your usual dishes. When you see that what you pour as a cereal bowl could actually amount to 2, 3, or even more servings, it will come as quite a surprise! Using your own plates and bowls to the size of various portions will help you cut back on the amount of food you consume and of caloric intake. Another trick is serving a normal portion of yourself, cutting half, and setting it aside as another meal.

TAKING DIETARY SUPPLEMENTS

A lot of people feel it is important to take dietary supplements in an attempt to improve strength, alleviate stress, and enhance physical health. Nonetheless, doctors believe, for the most part, that eating a well-balanced diet is all you need to fulfill your energy needs. For the exception of pregnant women and older

adults who can benefit from supplements like folic acid and vitamin C and calcium, respectively, your daily food intake will provide you with all you need.

New, organically produced whole foods that contribute to your wellbeing in three main ways:

1. Provide a wider variety of micronutrients to boost nutrition quality

2. Provide the dietary fiber necessary for healthy digestion

3. Provide additional compounds such as phytochemicals and antioxidants that work within the body to protect against a range of diseases such as cancer, heart disease, and diabetes

However, there are other experts who argue that even eating what is called a well-balanced diet is not enough because the food we eat comes from nutrient-poor soils or is picked early and

force-ripened. The way food is prepared can also decrease the nutrient value you 'd expect to receive. Canned and processed foods have lost much of their intrinsic nutritional value, and further cooking only further lowers the standard. Additionally, some of the highest concentrations of the nutritional value of the product are lost when the skins of fruits and vegetables are extracted.

So what should the public do? If you're worried about your health (and if you're reading this book, you have to be!), you should get the best advice from a nutritionist or your primary healthcare provider. Beyond a multi-vitamin and maybe a fiber supplement, various items can have unintended side effects for each other, or you might be taking prescription drugs. To prevent complications, let a doctor help with the decision to add some other dietary supplements to boost your physical and

mental health!

Protein supplements can be helpful for bodybuilders and hardcore athletes right after intense workouts. There should be adequate protein in the diet for anyone else, and if more protein is needed, it can come from adding some nuts, lean meat, a glass of skim or low-fat milk, or one of the many other sources of protein as a snack. Like for every supplement, protein powders and shakes are made from a number of sources and contain a variety of ingredients, most of which can be carbohydrates. Whey and casein, which come from plant-based milk and soy, are the best options.

Building muscle mass means eating more of the right kinds of foods, particularly those with high protein content. Lean, grass-fed beef, chicken, fish eggs, and dairy products are key protein sources, but there are other foods that play important roles in

muscle mass as a whole. Brown rice, quinoa, whole grains, and oatmeal offer a range of nutrients that contain important amino acids, help regulate the development of insulin, raise growth hormone levels, and make you stay full longer. Also quite important are fruits and vegetables, with apples, oranges, beets, spinach, and other dark green, leafy vegetables, tomatoes, and broccoli, among the most beneficial. Whey powder is a great supplement, and after a workout, can be used for a drink.

More often, eating smaller meals (or at least three moderate meals with three healthy snacks) is the ideal way to keep the body fuelled and provide all the essential nutrients for muscle growth and maintenance. Include a bit of protein in each of the six 'meals;' for mid-morning, and mid-afternoon snacks, some yogurt and berries, a protein powdered smoothie, low-fat milk, and berries or some fruit, whole wheat bread or crackers, and

peanut butter provide an energy boost and nutrition that creates muscle.

THE BODY REQUIRES PLENTY OF WATER

Water is the primary component of our bodies and should be periodically replenished. When the body sweats, fluid is lost very easily during strenuous exercise and must be replaced. This can add up to anywhere from 2 to 3 gallons for intense workouts!

Within the body, water has many essential functions:

- Helps regulate body temperature

- It adds fluid to the blood to facilitate oxygen and nutrient transport

- This flushes out toxins and cellular waste

- It increases the digestive cycle and operation of the kidneys.

Sports drinks are very popular, but there are those who believe that plain water is all the hydration needs of the body. This is generally accurate for most individuals who work at a modest pace for less than an hour, but there are benefits of consuming goods with added electrolytes and carbohydrates when there is heavy or long-lasting action.

In addition, too much water may be harmful in that it causes the kidneys to release excess fluid, and can result in dehydration. In sports drinks, sodium compensates for the salt lost by sweat and is important as it helps the body retain water and channels the fluids into the bloodstream and necessary muscles. Carbohydrates provide a simple source of energy for fatiguing cells, providing them with a boost to longer stamina.

Water is used for every process that the body performs, from the transportation of nutrients around the body to essential brain

functions. Most areas around the world have drinking water readily accessible, and there is really no reason to be dehydrated. A good tip is to take a bottle of water with you anywhere you go and often take small sips. It will ensure that anything you may be doing is still hydrated.

Just subtract your weight by 0.033 kg to figure out how much you will be drinking. I weigh 75 kg, for example, so 75 kg x 0.033 = 2.475 litres. So I should be aiming for 2.5 liters of water per day. If you live in a hot place, or you've trained hard, just drink more to make up for it.

Note: just divide your weight by 2.2 in pounds to bring your weight into pounds. 165lbs, for example, divided by 2.2 = 75 kg

Another word of caution about the type of drink you choose to hydrate: you should avoid drinking a sugar beverage because the sudden sugar flood is burned as fuel much easier than fat or

protein, but when the sugar is gone, the body takes a while to adjust to the change, leading to what is called a 'sugar crash.' Carbonated drinks should also be avoided due to the pain that the gas can cause and the risk of cramps and diarrhea forming.

BODY DETOXIFICATION

Detoxification is a trendy topic, with many pros and cons. Drastic measures such as colonic flushes or special diets with fasting periods are not considered to be really necessary, but the idea of helping the body remove toxins should be given attention. This is particularly true when starting a diet and exercise plan because many toxins are stored in fat. These toxins are released into the system when the fat is broken down, and this sudden rush can cause feelings of fatigue, muscle soreness, and even nausea. For improved functioning, a balanced diet and

increased metabolic activity due to exercise should keep the detoxification pathways open.

The body absorbs harmful substances in several ways:

- Digestive mode

- Kidneys (to the bladder, and urine removal)

- Headache (filters blood)

- Lymph nodes

- Air conditioning machine

- Skin (By sweat)

One way to make your diet more enjoyable and help with the detox process is by adding a range of herbs and spices. Digestion benefits from Anise, Basil, Burdock, Cilantro, Cinnamon, Cayenne, Cloves, Cumin, Garlic, Ginger, Ginseng, Licorice, Milk Thistle, Mint, Nutmeg, Oregano, Rosemary, Sage, Schizandra, Thyme, and Turmeric all.

To maintain a steady nutrient supply, it is recommended that you add some balanced snacks that include a small portion of lean protein or mid-morning and mid-afternoon nuts. Green tea is a healthier choice as compared to coffee, and adding a few lemon wedges or juice to water helps a large variety of body problems.

When you start a healthy lifestyle, it's getting easier and easier. A proper diet provides better physical function and more energy, so exercise is less of a challenge, and more exercise provides more energy and greater use of oxygen and nutrients, which leads to weight loss. You will continue to do the things that support that state of being when you feel good, so you are more likely to continue eating properly and exercising regularly.

PREPARE MEALS IN BULK

Anyone who has ever read any forums or magazines on bodybuilding or muscle and fitness should know this rule, which is to make food in bulk. The production of food in bulk serves several purposes:

Firstly, it means that a decent meal is always to be enjoyed whenever you're hungry.

Second, it allows you to take this food to work, gymnasium, train, etc., so you don't end up buying junk food when you're away from home. Also, preparing food in bulk takes less time, and it costs less money than cooking a single meal whenever you need to eat.

There's more than enough recipes out there to teach you how to cook in bulk, so I'm not going to bore you with all of them, but I'm suggesting nutrient-rich meals. I live in the U.K., for example, where the weather can often be cold and damp (OK, a

lot of the time), and I like to make stews, casseroles, soups and other hot meals for my bulk food. These contain lots of protein and healthy meat fats, lots of carbohydrates and other vegetable nutrients, and are fast and simple to eat and need no more preparation than heating it up in a microwave oven. Another very common idea is using plastic tubs to hold the food in. Personally, I've got lots of these lying around, both big ones I'm freezing in and smaller ones I 'm taking to work, train, travel, gym, and so on.

A SAMPLE DIET

To finish this portion, we'll look at a sample diet on any given day that's pretty typical of me. This is just an example, which serves to show how simple, easy, and cheap it can be to eat a very good diet that will help you build strength and performance in

athletics.

Breakfast

I have almost always scrambled an egg for breakfast. This consists of 2 to 3 eggs mixed with a small quantity of milk, then cooked to ready. At the same time, I also eat some fruit, most commonly a banana and an apple. I also combine this with lots of water or milk of good quality. Don't fall for the nonsense of low-fat milk; get the fatest, most healthy stuff you can find. You should try to build strength and not compete in a competition for fitness modeling.

Snack

I almost always eat a combination of unprocessed nuts, seeds, and dried fruit for snacks. Cashews, brazils, almonds, raisins, cranberries, and so on are in my mix today. So you get good

protein, fats, and carbohydrates with a snack that doesn't need any preparation. Again, there's good fruit here too, or even a small can of tuna or a chicken breast.

Lunch

My lunch is usually a meal that I prepared in bulk either the night before or a couple of days before. This can be tuna salad, chicken salad, stewed beef, vegetable roast chicken, etc. Be sure to have plenty of vegetables along with the source of protein, because this will give you plenty of nutrients your body requires.

Snack

My second snack is the same as before, but it can be added fruit or leftover during lunch.

Supper

Normally the last meal of the day is another bulk meal or can be made on the day. For example, with peanut butter and cream cheese sauce, sweet potatoes, peas, sweet corn, asparagus, and broccoli, I would have diced chicken breast.

CHAPTER SIX: REST AND RECOVERY

Contrary to common opinion, as you're running, the body isn't getting stronger or fitter. It gets better in the gaps between training sessions, and it has to be given a chance to heal for that to happen. The human body is an adaptive organism, and it can and will recover from almost anything given sufficient rest, proper nutrition, and adequate sleep. Within this segment, we will look at four areas, which are sleep, what to do if you get hurt, take care of your hands, and the strength of the tendon and the ligament.

THE TIME FOR REST

There's nothing more important about recovering from your workouts than adequate rest, good nutrition, and sleep above all else. Many people, at any rate, do not get close enough sleep anywhere in the modern world. There is good scientific evidence

to suggest that if your sleep is either too short, interrupted, or if you go to bed too late, the body will not repair itself anywhere near as effectively. Having a good night's sleep is something that these days, for many reasons, is becoming much rarer. Work tension, busy family life, financial problems, and many other factors can all add up to make it difficult to sleep a good night. I've had these issues, just like many of you might have read this, but there are a variety of things you can do to make sure you get a good night's rest:

Make sure you get to bed on time, first. This means you will be asleep by 22:30 pm at the latest. Everything later, and you're going to miss the valuable time your body is using to repair itself. Now I know it's not always easy to get to bed, let alone sleep, before 10:30 pm, but try to do it on the days and nights you do.

Secondly, keep your mobile phone and any other electronic

device off for at least twenty minutes before you go to bed. The screen's bright light and glare won't do your eyes any good, and the electrical and magnetic field generated by those devices can't be good for your brain as it attempts to shut down. There is some research in this area, but because most people are more or less addicted to checking their social media accounts before turning in, it has not received much attention. By the end of the day, if you are serious about having real strength from Calisthenics, then your status report can wait until the morning.

Thirdly, if there are things you 're concerned about, such as a variety of things you'll have to do the next day, then write them down in a little notepad that you'll keep at your bedside. I started doing this a long time ago, and it is extremely helpful. If you have thousands of thoughts and ideas bouncing up there like me, the best thing you need to do is get them out and write them

down. I noticed that in a sense, this almost puts them away, so my mind can be calm, and I still sleep better because of it.

Third, make your bedroom as dark as it can be. The darker the room, the easier it will be for you to shut down and get to sleep faster, this is a no brainer. Attempt to get dark-colored curtains over your current curtains or blinds, or drape a towel or something else.

Eventually, try to learn to meditate. OK, I'm not a spiritualist, and I don't believe in any new age theory, but in the modern world, the ability to shut down thoughts and brain is very rare and can be incredibly helpful to those of you who still struggle to sleep even after all the measures listed above.

INJURY AND CALISTHENICS

Although there is little chance of getting injured while

performing Calisthenics, the more advanced exercises do place a great deal of stress and strain on the bones, muscles, tendons, and ligaments of the body, so the chance and risk of injury is never totally nil. There are things that you can do to avoid getting hurt, like no overtraining, only improving when you're ready, and above all, giving your body enough time to adjust to the demands put on it. Also, ensure that the mobility and flexibility exercises discussed and illustrated in the previous chapters are followed, as this will help to address and avoid any potential problems. If you get injured, then rest and seek professional advice is the best thing to do. I've had some physiotherapist experience, and while there are some who aren't really good at all, there are people out there who have the skills to help with sports and strength-related training injuries. The most common niggles and injuries you may encounter in your own training are unique to Calisthenics, and a few of them are

worth talking about here, just so you know what to look for and what to do if you succumb to them.

Firstly, since the elbow joint is extensively used in Calisthenics, the risk of tendonitis is slight. Planks, front levers, back levers, and human flags are all done with straight arms, and although this is not in and of itself harmful, overuse can occur, and the elbow joint can become very painful and inflexible. The same will happen while practicing for one-arm pull-ups and other movements that place a lot of pressure on the upper body joints' ligaments and tendons. This is why I recommend keeping the repetition ranges low on movements such as the one-arm pull-up and other similar exercises, as I explain in the exercise section.

Second, in almost all calisthenics exercises, the core takes a huge pounding, so watch out for soreness and any stresses and strains there. I have overdone it a few times in my own preparation and

pulled my muscles, so much so that it was hard to get out of bed for about a week. If this is the case again, then the solution will be more rest and less training time. Any serious injury, like a hernia, needs to be treated by a qualified medical practitioner and seen.

Third, the shoulders are the one joint that is likely to come under the most stress during the training in Calisthenics. That is because the scapula is by far the most unstable joint in the body. This means that the risk of injury is higher here than in many other areas of the body, and that is why I suggest performing appropriate warm-ups and exercises on mobility. You'll be exposed to scapula strengthening movements in the next segment, PART III, which can help create nearly bombproof shoulders. If you have long been serious about training and don't want to get injured, make sure you do them.

Finally, the hands will be active in virtually all the exercises included in this book and in all the movements of Calisthenics, and as such, will be put under tremendous stress and pressure while you work. Make sure you stretch them out before and after your session, and if you feel any unusual pain in them at all, then stop the exercise and let them rest. In the next section, I talk more extensively about hand care.

HOW TO TAKE CARE OF YOUR HANDS

For all the parts of the body involved in Calisthenics, as I have already explained, the one that is most used is without question the hands. The hands are used heavily for virtually every workout, including pushing, pulling, and many of the core exercises, and can really take a beating. It 's critical that we look after them in that regard. We will look after the hands in the

same way as we do mobility and strengthening exercises for the feet, and conduct stability drills for the entire body.

The first thing you will find when you start calisthenics training is that the palms of the hands can be very sore, particularly after a hard pull-up session, or after an extended period of time using the parallets. It is a common and natural response on the part of the body, and there is nothing you can do to prevent soreness, except rest and maybe moisturize. Do NOT be tempted to use gloves. It will only create more issues later, particularly when it's time to start learning the wrong grip and other movements in the hands that require full sensitivity and feeling.

The second thing that will happen is that the body will develop calluses in reaction to the soreness and the use of hands, most commonly where the fingers touch the palm and on each of the finger joints themselves. That's usual again, but you shouldn't let

them get too high, as these also have the negative impact of getting stuck on stuff and getting in the way when you catch a pull-up bar or other item. These will also pile up and pinch every time the hand is closed into a fist, which can be painful once again. The only remedy I've found is to sand down and raising the callus height to the point that they're still there, but not completely gone. For this job, you can use a range of devices, including nail files, very light sandpaper, and some beauty items designed to get rid of dry and dead skin. For a variety of reasons, this is important; the main ones are that the skin is hardening in certain places for a reason, and you need that to avoid blisters and other rips and tears from occurring. Getting broken hands can sound large and smart, and not a week goes by where I don't see an image of someone's bleeding hands proudly posted on the internet, but the most that can do is only give you a few weeks off training, which isn't an ideal situation if you're trying to

make progress and get stronger.

Last but not least, if you use some sort of chalk in your workout, and particularly if you use liquid chalk, then after every workout, your hands will definitely need moisturizer. The alcohol in liquid chalk will absolutely dry out your palms, leaving them more vulnerable to damage from rips and falls, so make sure you do that, no matter how un-macho it can seem. It's a lot more un-macho to have to take some time off training because you didn't take two minutes to look after your face.

TENDON STRENGTH AND LIGAMENT

The last part of this segment deals with the strength of tendon and ligament, and the ways it varies from muscle strength. While muscles are responsible for moving the joints, and hence

all human activity, the tendons and ligaments bind the muscle to the bone and that bone to bone. A part of strength training that is often ignored or overlooked in general is that all areas of the body take the same time to heal and recover. This is not true and is particularly important in our case, as calisthenics training relies heavily on the strength of the tendons and ligaments. If we take the planche example, there is a height of force that must be transmitted through the tendon of the biceps and the other connective tissues in order to complete the motion. When you don't give enough time to repair these issues, then you won't recover in time, and you won't get stronger.

Estimates vary, but tendons and ligaments take up to ten times as long to heal for the average person if they are injured as the muscles that surround them. It means that if the muscles take three days to recover from a sprain or strain, then it will take 30

days for the tendon or ligament! If you experience pain in your elbows or some other place due to muscle soreness, then relax. Don't be tempted to push your luck, because the only thing that's going to happen is that you're going to hurt yourself even more and that's going to set you back weeks or months.

CHAPTER SEVEN: PHYSICAL PREPARATION -1

In this section, we will look at a variety of very critical training pieces that are often totally ignored by a lot of people. They include warming up, stability, training for exercises, and versatility. If you want to progress quickly and without injury, all these stages are vital, and I would encourage you to read and absorb as much of it as possible.

WARM-UP

Warming up before any workout is a good idea, but if you are going to train using Calisthenics, it is even more important. The amount of muscle used and the strength of these muscle contractions make it a must to make sure you 're completely warm and prepared before you start your workout. This is not to

say that every warm-up exercise known to man has to be spent hours going through. Some people spend far too long warming up in my experience, at the cost of actually exercising, and see poor results because they simply don't spend enough time actively performing the movements that lead to improvements in power. Additionally, if you spend too long or spend too much warming up, there is a chance you won't be able to put as much effort into your actual workout. This is a big mistake because you want to try and get as much out of every session as you can.

The first part of the warm-up has to be a cardiovascular variety in order to regulate and supple the body temperature and the muscles, tendons, and ligaments. This may be something you want, but there are a variety of items that work better than others. Running or jogging is the simplest, since it needs no equipment and can be done even in a relatively small area. If you

have access to a gym, then there is very nice cardiovascular equipment for the initial heating up. All good pieces of equipment for raising the body temperature and increasing the heart rate are the bike, rowing machine, and cross trainer or elliptical. The amount of time you'll need to do this for depends entirely on the person, but usually five to eight minutes is long enough for most people to feel warm and ready for their workout. Whichever form you use, as long as you feel at the end of the workout physically and mentally comfortable, that is sufficient.

MOBILITY

Once you've warmed up to a good level and feel warm and ready to start, it's recommended that you do some work on mobility before starting your workout properly. Mobility can be loosely

defined as the ability of the body to shift into positions under the power of its own muscles. Mobility shortages can seriously hamper your progress as being unable to get into the correct body positions will not allow you to exert as much force in the exercise and limit your gains in strength.

In the years I've been researching training methods and programming, mobility itself has become much more normal and widespread, and it's very unusual these days to find any competitor who either doesn't do it or doesn't think it's beneficial. It can also help relieve muscle pain and soreness, get rid of any knots and tight areas, and simply keep all running properly.

I've divided the mobility exercises into three parts: upper body mobility, heart or torso mobility, and lower body movement. Ideally, these exercises should be completed at the beginning of

each workout, but this is not completely necessary. Mobility is one of those odd things which the less you need to do, the more you do. It may sound counterintuitive, but if you've got good durability, you'll have to spend much less time sustaining it than you had it first.

You would simply need to get into a certain body position for some of the mobility movements or shift into a certain position and out of it again, but for others, you will need access to a foam roller, as stated in the equipment section.

UPPER BODY MOBILITY

Upper body mobility, especially the hamstrings, is often neglected in favor of spending time on the lower body. In most people, the hamstrings are strong, which is maybe why they are

spending so much time stretching them out. However, in order to be able to transfer power and deal with physical situations that arise in any sport, upper body flexibility, and mobility, especially in the shoulder-girdle, is very important. Bad mobility here will also stop you from entering positions like the handstand and, in the long run, will just hinder you.

SCAPULA MOVEMENT

The first few mobility exercises we'll be looking at are the scapula ones I first mentioned in the introductory section. These are the push-up scapula, scapula lines, scapula dive, pull-up scapula, and pull-up scapula with one-arm. These are designed to strengthen and maximize the stability of the entire shoulder girdle and have long been a staple of my training.

SCAPULA PUSH-UPS

Scapula push-ups are an important exercise and can be very helpful when training for the planche and some of the other levers, such as the front lever and back lever. This can be thought of as a 'pushing' scapula exercise, and it is again effective in floor movements such as the planche and various levers.

1. Position yourself in a push-up position with a neutral posture to push the scapula up.

2. Lower your chest down to the floor from here, and squeeze your scapula together as you do. Do NOT bend the elbows.

3. Reverse the movement once you reach the bottom position, so that your shoulder blades separate and your spine rises. Keep pushing until it circles your back, and your spine is as high as

possible. Do NOT bend the elbows during motion at any point.

Repeat for ten repetitions.

SCAPULA DIPS

The second movement driving scapula is the dip of the scapula. In fact, this really should be called the reverse scapula shrug, as it is the opposite step to a conventional shrug, but no matter. Each exercise is meant to reinforce the shoulders for activities such as handstands, planks, and other exercises based on floors.

1. Place yourself in the top part of a Triceps dip to do scapula dips. Maintain a neutral body.

2. Let your entire body fall from here so that your shoulders rise to reach your ears. Keep your elbows locked all along.

3. Push up vigorously from this bottom point, trying to push the

whole body as far as possible down into the air and the shoulders. Do NOT curl your elbows anywhere. Repeat for ten repetitions.

SCAPULA PULL-UP

Some of the most important exercises that we can use to improve scapula force are what I call the pull-up scapula. You grow an immense amount of strength when you work efficiently with the entire body weight.

1. Take a pull-up bar with an overhand grip to perform scapula pull-ups, and hang with completely straight arms.

2. Make sure the scapula's lifted. It would be whether the shoulders are close to or touching the face, as seen in the following images.

3. Try to pull your scapula down from this dead hanging position, Just bending your elbows. What can sound difficult to do at first, but persevere before you do. The range of motion you'll achieve depends on a variety of factors, including your strength, endurance, and physiology of the arm.

4. Keep this position for a second after you have pulled your scapula down, then drop back to the start spot. Repeat for ten reps. With this move, you can use weight to great effect, too.

SCAPULA ONE-ARM PULL-UP

When you've become familiar with the pull-up scapula, you should try moving on to the one-armed version. This variation would be invaluable in learning one arm chin-ups, as one of the toughest (if not the toughest) aspects of the one arm chin-up is

having the pull started from the dead hanging position. The part becomes much easier as the strength of the scapula increases.

1. To pull-up, the one-armed scapula, catch a pull-up bar in an overhand or underhand grip with one hand and hang with a fully locked arm. You can put the other arm wherever you want, but I'd rather have it crossed over my chest or before my torso.

2. Make sure the scapula's lifted. It would be while your ear is close or touching your head, as seen in the following images.

3. Attempt to pull your scapula down from this dead hanging spot FOR bending your elbow. What can sound difficult to do at first, but persevere before you do. The range of motion you'll achieve depends on a variety of

factors, including your strength, endurance, and physiology of the arm.

4. Keep this position for a few seconds after you have pulled your scapula down and then drop back to the starting spot. Repeat on each Arm for five reps.

SCAPULA FOAM ROLLING

In addition to actually exercising and strengthening the scapulas, it is necessary to roll them on foam, particularly if you have any tight areas or sore bits or knots within the muscle, as this will significantly help to improve mobility in this region.

1. You place yourself on top of the foam roller to foam the scapulas and then placed your body in a hollow place. To do so, hug yourself, in order to round your back.

2. Now over the foam roller roll back and forth, stopping and going slowly when you encounter some sore points. Spend about 20 to 30 seconds doing this.

ARMPIT FOAM ROLLING

One place where most of the people are close is the armpits and shoulders. This is a consequence of the modern world, where many people spend hours each day either sitting at a desk or driving, shortening and tightening the muscles in the front of the body, and stretching and weakening those in the back. We can fix this by rolling foam on some areas, and we will foam the axle for this versatility drill.

1. Lay face down and place the foam roller to the body at ninety degrees to foam roll the armpit. Extend your arm over your head and place your axle right atop the roller.

2. Then roll forward and backward ten times, slowly rolling gradually over the sore sections and letting the roller do its job. Then move across and repeat.

ROTATOR CUFF STRETCH

The musculature of the rotator cuff is responsible for several shoulder movements, and should, therefore, be spread out prior to any activity involving the shoulders.

1. Lying on one side flat on the field to stretch the rotator cuff muscles. Place your left arm out to your body at 90 degrees, with your hand pointed up into the air.

2. Use your right hand to grab your left wrist and start pushing it gently down towards the ground. Keep the 90-

degree bend in your elbow, and continue to apply pressure while keeping your left shoulder on the ground. Keep the stretch, change arms, and repeat for 30 seconds.

CHEST AND SHOULDER STRETCH

It is really important to open the chest and shoulders before we start a training session, and this next stretch is one of the best in terms of stretching out and moving the back, armpits, and chest.

1. Find a space on the ground to stretch the shoulder and arms, and get on your hands and knees.

2. Now lift your hips into the air, as seen in the photo, and lower your chest towards the bottom. Keep thinking about pulling down the shoulders and chest to increase

the stretch through the ground. Keep this, and release for around 15 to 20 seconds.

SHOULDER DISLOCATES

The last segment of our upper body mobility drills is shoulder dislocates. Don't worry, your shoulders won't dislocate, but if you've got tight shoulders or weak strength in your upper body, you'll really feel them. You will need some kind of bar to perform them, preferably one which is very light. Broom handles are excellent for this movement, or exercise class barbells.

1. To dislocate your shoulder, stand apart with your feet shoulder-width and hold the bar with an overhand grip in front of you. Start with a grip as wide as you can. Starting here, push the bar up in a wide arc above your

head and finish with the bar resting on your lower back.

Ensure you are still keeping your elbows straight.

Perform two sets of 10 repetitions with the rest of around

20 to 30 seconds in between.

2. When you're struggling to get the movement done at all,

    try pushing your hands farther apart before you can. As

    your shoulders become more flexible, just move the

    hands closer together to make the movement more

    difficult. The pictures below thoroughly display the

    movement.

CHAPTER EIGHT: PHYSICAL PREPARATION - 2

CORE AND LOWER BODY MOBILITY

Core mobility is somewhat less extensive than upper body or lower body mobility, mainly because the heart can not move as

much as the upper body and lower body, and the spine is not really capable of a wide variety of motions. How ever, keeping and maintaining mobility here is still important to you, as you do not want to be limited in your movements due to lack of flexibility in the spine.

SPINE ROLLING-FOAM

As mentioned in the book's earlier section, foam rolling is a helpful addition to a mobility routine and can help relieve some injury issues or lack of mobility. Foam rolling the spine is good for a number of things; firstly, it can help to reduce the number of knots and tight areas in the back, in particular muscle groups, and secondly, it can improve the spine's extending capability.

1. Place a foam roller ninety degrees into your chest to shake the

spine and put your lower back on it. Hold your feet on the floor, and get your hands ready to help if you need it.

2. Move back and forth over the roller, starting from the base of the spine, slowing down on any sore parts and paying careful attention to them. Continue until you hit the back top where you can stop and try to let your spine curl around the roller. This will help stretch the chest and increase the strength and flexibility of the upper back.

SIDE LEANS

The obliques are one part of the heart that is particularly disturbing for many people. They are the muscles in the torso sides, and they are responsible for helping you to bend sideways to the waist. The lower part of your spine will also dictate how flexible you are going to be here, so this is important for those with low spinal flexibility levels as well.

- You will need a bar or rod of some kind to perform side leans, preferably the same type that you used for dislocating the shoulder. Stand wide apart with your feet and grip the bar in both hands, roughly as wide as your feet are so that your whole body forms a broad "X" shape.

- Bend over to one side at the waist from here, using the muscles at the sides of your core. Keep your arms straight at all times, and don't allow your shoulders to move towards your head; the movement just has to come from your waist.

- Adjust to the upright position once you have gotten as low as you can, and repeat on the other leg. Repeat so for every ten repetitions.

THE LOWER BODY MOBILITY

The lower body is used as a mode of transportation all the time, even if you don't train or participate in any sporting activity, so it's usually home to many mobility issues, especially if you've never taken the time to prepare for workouts or stretch afterward. This usually manifests itself later in mobility and performance issues and can be difficult to correct once it reaches that stage. Fortunately, it is very easy to boost and retain lower body mobility. The movements and agility drills that I mentioned in this next section should be done for better results every day, preferably before your training starts, and also on rest days to keep things going properly. The specific movements themselves are based on stretches and movement of foam rolling that have been part of the strength and conditioning programs for a long time now, with additional feedback from Joe DeFranco from DeFranco's gym in the USA. There are several different exercises that you can do for mobility, but these are the

exercises that I consider to be the most effective and that I use very frequently.

THE FOAM ROLLING BAND

Foam rolling band is the first part of our lower body training. Of this part of the anatomy, the proper name is the iliotibial band, which is a long tendon that stretches from the hip to the knee joint down the outside of the leg. This area, particularly in runners, is prone to getting very tight and can cause multiple knee problems.

1. Lay flat on one side to pad the IT band, and the top of the leg lies on a roller. Then turn back and forth until there are sore spots around the outside of the leg. Make sure to roll all the way down from your hip to the knee joint. Spend rolling on each leg

for 15 seconds or more.

THE FOAM ROLLING ADDUCTOR

The adductors play their part in hip drive and power generation in the lower body along with the hamstrings and the glutes, so it is vital to have the mobile and unhindered.

1. You put the roller on the ground at ninety degrees to your body to foam the adductors, putting the inside of the thigh against it. Now roll forward, to the hip itself from the inside of the thigh. Spend rolling on each leg for 15 seconds or more.

FOAM ROLLING PIRIFORMIS

As you begin to incorporate more squatting and hip movements into your workout, you may find the piriformis, or the muscle on the outside of the hip, becoming very tight. The best way of counteracting this is to roll the piriformis with some sort of ball, preferably one that is hard enough to get into the muscle. With a tennis ball, you can start and progress on tougher and harder balls.

1. Sit down and place your right foot on your left knee to roll the piriformis, as if you'd cross your legs. Now sit with the piriformis straight on the ball. You 're going to know if you're in the right place because it's going to feel sore and tender. Roll over the tight spot slowly, or just sit on the tender spot and let the ball sink into the muscle, making sure to spend more time on the sorest area. Then turn the legs and repeat.

2. When the piriformis has been rolled, you can do static stretching. To do so, sit on a bench at ninety degrees with your right foot flat on the floor and knee. Place your left foot over your right knee and move your knee down. You'll feel the stretch in the glute leg. Seek to keep your head straight and take a deep breath. Hold the stretch for 15 seconds, then swap sides and repeat again.

STRADDLE ROLLOVERS

In many areas of the lower body, rollers generate mobility and flexibility, including the glutes, hamstrings, groin, and the hip area in general. We need a bit of flexibility in the hips, and they only do as much as they can.

1. Place the legs in front of you to execute the rollovers.

2. Now turn back onto your back and throwback your legs.

3. Now push yourself up again to a seated position, but spread your legs in a wide straddle. When you do so, stretch as far as possible between your thighs. It is known to be a repeat. Allow ten repetitions of the workout.

FIRE HYDRANTS

Fire hydrants are another very great exercise in lower body mobility, which helps to open the hips and prepare them for lower body movement.

1. You put yourself on your hand and knees to conduct fire hydrants.

2. Lift one leg up to the side from here, stretch the knee backward and then push it forward as far as you can

before bringing it on the floor again. This exercise is aimed at drawing a very wide arc with the knee. Perform the movement on each leg ten times forward and ten times backward.

MOUNTAIN CLIMBERS

Mountain climbers are excellent conditioning and metabolism that increase exercise, and they can also help build more mobility in the hips with a slight alteration. In this cycle, you can get a healthy hip flexor and hamstring stretch too.

1. To do mountain climbers, get in a push-up position with one leg spread out behind you and the other positioned as near as possible to the side of your chest.

2. Holding the arms straight, hop both feet into the air and turn

them over, so the back foot gets to the front, and the front foot goes backward. Repeat for ten reps.

FROG HOPS

Frog hops are a variation of mountain climbers requiring more flexibility because both feet will move to the sides of the hands. Make sure you jump the two feet wide, so your legs don't knock into your arms.

1. Get in a push-up position to perform frog hops.

2. From here, leap both feet forward until you hit the outside of your legs, then jump back to the push-up position once more. This will require good hip mobility, so just keep working with them until the location shown

in the following pictures is reachable. Perform 10 of those repetitions.

CHAPTER NINE: CALISTHENICS AND FLEXIBILITY EXERCISES

Now that we've looked at a variety of mobility exercises that you can do to enhance that part of your performance, versatility is the next thing to analyze. Flexibility is the strength of your muscles to allow your joints to shift into any place unhindered, and the main trouble areas for calisthenics are the shoulders and hips. Flexibility is perhaps the most overlooked aspect of preparation for the majority of people. Following their workout, aside from a few fast stretches, most of us never spend any time trying to develop our versatility. It's vital to avoid injury, to stay active as we get older, to increase recovery rates, and to perform some of the more challenging exercises in this book. While a full

guide to versatility is beyond this volume 's reach, the stretches I have provided will still yield many benefits. If you want to find out more about versatility, then there are a lot of interesting books out there. "Relax into Stretch," by Pavel Tsatsouline, is one of my favorites.

These are a variety of body areas that we will be paying attention to, and these are discussed next.

In terms of the upper body, most people have strong muscles at the front of the body and weak and lose muscles at the back of the body during these days of driving and computing and office work. This can be easily illustrated in the posture of almost anyone you see; broad shoulders and a forward jutting head, and their reluctance to lift their arms above the head. It takes a little time to fix this issue, but the effort is well worth it.

For other men, too, the lower body involves other issues. The

hips can be thought of as the body's hinge, and if the areas around the hips are not flexible, then some of the exercises in this book can cause you real trouble. There can be a lack of flexibility in this area due to a variety of reasons, but more often than not, due to tightness in the hamstrings, adductors or groin, and piriformis. Luckily, these things are easy to deal with, and once you have achieved the degree of versatility and agility you need, it can be retained with little effort.

A common misconception about flexibility is that it is limited by the muscle's physical shortness. That's not real. Flexibility, or the lengthening capacity of your muscles, is controlled by your nervous system and is not really "stretching" because of your muscles. It is the stretch reflex firing that stops you from going any further when you reach the limit of your flexibility. In order to become more resilient, we need to re-educate our nervous

system so that our muscles can achieve their maximum capacity.

There are many ways we can do that, but I've picked and outlined three of the best ways below.

You just have to relax

To increase your flexibility, you need to be relaxed. If you're tense, anxious, or uncomfortable, then you won't increase your flexibility. There are many ways to promote relaxation, but contrasting your breathing is one of the easiest and best methods.

Get into one stretch of your choice to do this. Expand the stretch until you reach your limit. Keep on for about 10 seconds before taking a deep breath. Keep this breath for a few seconds, and then release it in one go. Seek to make your whole body

relax as you do this. Your stretch should be getting longer. Repeat 3 to 5 times this cycle.

Make a lengthened muscle stronger

Perhaps the best way to increase your flexibility is to increase your muscle strength when stretching in a relaxed position. If a muscle is stronger in a lengthened position, it is much more likely that the nervous system will allow the body to get to that position first.

Simply assume a stretch position of your choosing to increase the strength of a stretched muscle. From here, the stretched muscles

contract while staying in the stretched position. Keep the contraction before relaxing for 5 to 10 seconds, and increasing the stretch. This can be replicated two or three times before the majority of people hit their limit. You can combine the two above strategies for better results to improve your versatility by a very significant amount.

Stick to it

As with anything in life, stretching every day for 10 minutes is much better than 2 hours once a month. Consistency can help improve and re-educate your nervous system to enable you to become more versatile.

THE STRETCHING GUIDE

You'll want to stretch after every workout, to begin with. This prevents the muscles from being too tight and preserves the strength you already have. To increase your flexibility by a large amount, you'll need to spend some time just stretching. A moderate stretching session of 20 to 30 minutes once a week is more than enough for most beginners. You 're probably going to feel very sore after that, but that's natural. When you become more versatile, and as your body learns to cope with the demands you put on it, you can gradually increase the number of stretching sessions you perform in a week. If you feel stiff and sore most of the time, you stretch too hard or too often. If this happens, simply the speed or volume of stretching you 're doing.

After a while, you will eventually achieve the amount of versatility you wish or need to do the exercises you use. When this happens, you should avoid trying to further increase your

versatility and instead concentrate on maintaining your current level of flexibility. How long you'll need to spend stretching to maintain that level depends on the individual, so you'll just have experimentation and find out. Most commonly, it takes far less time to maintain your flexibility than becoming really flexible in the first place.

UPPER BODY STRETCHES

The upper body is an important part of calisthenics and is used in most of the calisthenic exercises. To that end, exercising your upper body is a crucial part of your workout. Such stretches are to be done after your workout but can be done before or during your session if you feel tight in a certain area or if you need a little more movement before a specific exercise.

CHEST AND SHOULDER STRETCHES

The first stretch in this section is both a stretch of the shoulder and a stretch of the arm, which is exactly the same as the one we discussed in the section on mobility.

1. Find a space on the ground to stretch the chest and shoulder, and get on your hands and knees.

2. Now push your hips into the air, as shown in the picture, and move your chest towards the ground. Keep talking about pushing down the shoulders and chest to improve the stretch through the field. Hold this and release it for about 15 to 20 seconds.

UPPER BACK STRETCH

When you get to the harder pulling exercises, your back will be under a lot of stress, so relaxing this part of the body is vital to prevent any complications that might arise. This particular stretch puts a priority on the lattisimus dorsi or the broad wing as the back muscles.

1. Grab a strong surface with one arm and lean back to execute this move, holding your arm and legs straight.

2. Open your shoulder blades and squeeze your shoulders forward together. Across the gap, reach your opposite arm to increase the stretch. Hold that position for between 15 and 20 seconds.

CHEST STRETCH

Because many calisthenic exercises use a "hollow body" pose,

where the shoulders are rounded and the chest tensioned, it is important to stretch this area to ensure that you don't get too tight.

1. Place your palm against a solid object, like a wall or doorframe, to stretch the chest.

2. Hold your arm straight and turn your hand away before you feel the stretch. Keep this place, turn sides, and repeat for 15 seconds.

FOREARM AND WRIST STRETCH -1

Many of the handstands and pressing exercises are highly taxing on the wrists, so you might want to stretch them out before and after your workout. There are two main stretches of the wrist, and this is the first of them.

1. Place yourself on your hands and knees and place your hands with your fingers pointing upwards to perform the first wrist stretch.

2. Hold the arms straight, lean forward, and try to keep the palms pressed into the wall. Keep for 15 seconds this place.

FOREARM AND WRIST STRETCH -2

The second wrist stretch targets the forearm's upper side and is particularly useful following handstands and other similar exercises.

1. Position yourself on your hands and knees to perform this stretch and place your hands on the ground with your palms facing upwards.

2. Point your fingers back to your body and hold your arms straight until you feel the stretch. Hold on for 15 seconds with this location.

CORE STRETCHES

This is not only in the core exercises where the core muscles are used but also in movements of the upper body, such as the front lever and pull-up. That means stretching the core is very necessary if you want to remain mobile and flexible around the spine. However, since the core muscles are not so flexible and the torso is not capable of moving as much as other parts of the body, there will always be a somewhat limited range of motion here.

STANDING SIDE STRETCH

It is necessary to keep the sides of your torso flexible in order to allow you to perform the movements that require flexibility in the spine, and the standing side stretch will help to improve flexibility here.

1. Stand with your feet shoulder-width apart to extend the sides of your neck or obliques. Place one hand on your leg side and then reach overhead with the other hand.

2. Bend at the hip, simultaneously slip your hands down your leg and overhead, until you feel the stretch. Hold this position, change sides, and repeat for 15 seconds.

COBRA STRETCH

The cobra stretch is perfect for the rectus abdominis or six-pack,

and after dishes, half levers, and other core exercises, it can help alleviate cramp or soreness.

1. Lying face down on the floor with your hands flat to carry out the cobra stretch. Move your arms up, keeping your hands in contact with the bottom.

2. Curl the neck and look to the ceiling until the stretch is felt. Breathing deep inside and out in this position can help to increase the stretch. Hold on for 15 seconds with this position.

CAT STRETCH

Another effective movement taken from yoga is the cat stretch, which is perfect for targeting the middle, which lower back. This will also help t teach the shoulder blade separation that is

required in some of the other exercises of strength.

1. Position yourself on your hands and knees and push your spine up to the ceiling to perform the cat stretch.

2. Squeeze your shoulders together, and try to separate your shoulder blades. Hold on for 15 seconds with this position.

LOWER BODY STRETCHES

In this segment, we'll look at the stretches we can use to make the lower body more flexible. One of the most important things is flexibility in the lower body, as it's very easy to lose mobility and flexibility in the lower body as you get older. It can also help you to more easily perform the moves in the exercise section. For example, if you build flexibility in the hips, then it becomes

much easier to perform a movement like a straddle Blanche, as you will be able to perform a wider straddle, making it a little easier to hold the position of the planche, making your progress faster.

QUAD STRETCH

Nearly all lower-body movements include the quads or the front of the upper leg. Stretching them out is vital for maintaining proper function in the lower body.

1. Stand on one knee to stretch your quads (the front of your thigh) with something solid to hang on to.

2. Take the other foot, and pull the heel to the bum. Make sure you have your knees close together and push your

hips forward. Hold this position, change sides, and repeat for 15 seconds.

THE HAMSTRING STRETCH

The hamstrings, or the upper leg backs, are again engaged in almost all lower-body movements. They are also particularly susceptible to being tight in the vast majority of people, which is why you may want to spend more time stretching them out in the body than the other muscle groups.

1. Sit down and stretch one leg in front of you to reach your hamstrings, with the toe pointed towards the ceiling.

2. Put your other foot in the side of your leg and keep your arm forward, and try to touch your feet. Try to keep your

back straight from the hips and fold. Hold this position, change sides, and repeat for 15 seconds.

STRADDLE STRETCH

The seated straddle stretch is very useful for opening the hip joint and making the lower body more flexible. This stretch, once again, will help with movements and exercises like the planche.

1. Get into a seated position with your legs in the broadest "V" position you can manage to do the straddle stretch. Point your toes and fold at the knees until you feel the stretch.

2. With a partner, the stretch is also very successful. Get them to move your back halfway to increase the stretch. Hold on for 15 seconds with this position.

GROINS STRETCH

The groin, or adductor muscles, allow the hips to be more open and flexible, so we can use the seated groin stretch here to improve flexibility.

1. Sit down with your feet's soles together to execute this stretch, and draw them in as close to your butt as possible.

2. Stand up straight and try to keep your knees as low as you can to the floor. You can use the muscles on the outsides of your legs to pull down the thighs, or you can

simply place your arms or hands on them. Hold on for 15 seconds with this position.

HIP FLEXOR STRETCH

The hip flexors of most people are tight, and that may prevent the glutes from doing their job. Your jump and other lower body movements should improve after you have increased flexibility in your hip flexor.

1. Move into a kneeling posture with one leg in front of you to perform the hip flexor stretch. Hold the body straight and lean forward.

2. Around the top of your rear leg, you can experience a stretch. If you don't, then just increase the distance

between your knee and your foot. Hold this position,

change sides, and repeat for 15 seconds.

THE GLUTE STRETCH

The glutes, or bum muscles, are the body 's largest and most strong, so stretching them is necessary to maintain strength in running, jumping, and other lower body movements.

1. Sit down with one leg straight to execute the stretch, and the other leg tucked away, with the knee of the straight leg at the top of your foot.

2. Push the bent knee towards the right leg until the stretch in your glute is felt. Hold this position, change sides, and repeat for 15 seconds.

CALF STRETCH

The calves, or the lower leg bottom, are responsible for pointing the toes, and for foot balance and stability. They can also inhibit the body's ability to get into a deep squat position if they are tight.

1. Stand with your feet together and put your hands on a wall or other strong surface to perform the calf stretch.

2. Hold your legs straight on the table and your feet. Lean forwards until the stretch is felt. Hold on for 15 seconds with this position.

MORE FACTORS

We will look at other pieces of knowledge in this segment that we need to remember before going on and actually to look at the

exercises themselves. They are about the actual exercise results. We'll look at the range of motion in this segment, using momentum and cheating on the exercises.

RANGE OF MOTION

Range of motion, also abbreviated to ROM, refers to the maximum amount of movement that your joints in a particular exercise are capable of taking. For example, if we take the push-up, the full range of movement with the hands on the floor will include beginning with arms locked out, and then lowering down until the chest touches the floor. A reduced motion range would involve only a small amount of bending of the elbows, say until they reached 90 degrees. There are a number of reasons why the range of motion is important:

Firstly, the greater the range of motion, the easier the exercise will be, which will make you stronger in turn, with any exercise

requiring joint coordination, that is the case. Mobility and versatility can, of course, also decide how much motion you can obtain with such workouts, but as with all preparation, experience, and perseverance, all of these attributes can improve.

Secondly, the range of motion is necessary if the exercises are to be carried out properly. If we take the pull-up as another example, the hardest part of the movement is to get the elbows to bend in the pull from a dead hang where the arms are perfectly straight. If you do pull-ups and never lower yourself until your arms are straight, that part of the movement will still be heavy, regardless of how hard you exercise the rest of the movement.

Often an exercise with a maximum range of motion is not necessary since you may not be strong enough to complete the movement. For e.g., you can not be powerful enough to move

from the bottom position while learning the triceps dip. In such

cases, operating with a reduced ROM is just fine to the point

that you are strong enough to execute the movement properly.

CHAPTER TEN: ESSENTIAL EXERCISES IN CALISTHENICS

When done the right way, workouts involving calisthenics and bodyweight will help you accomplish almost every fitness goal. This has been how it has been done for thousands of years, after all! The important thing to realize is that it's not necessarily how many reps or sets you can do as much as the accuracy you 're doing them with. Just like keeping the tires balanced on the vehicle, the muscles work for their optimum efficiency by using the correct form.

A key element in the proper performance of calisthenics is the capacity of the body to travel through space in a manner under pressure. In the joints, there are receptors as well as the sense of balance in the inner ear that helps us distinguish where our body parts are in relation to each other and the ground. Learning how

to do an exercise properly and practicing the action over and over helps train the CNS. It allows for automated synchronization of all flexing and relaxing muscles. That is how a pitcher in baseball perfects a pitch, or a golfer masters a putt.

The perfecting of the steps of these basic exercises helps everyone to prepare for advanced sports, improved strength, and well-defined muscle mass beyond merely exercising for general health and weight loss.

BEGIN WITH THE BASICS

Though there are literally hundreds of different options that qualify as calisthenics or exercises on body weight, the basics are where they all start. Here are 12 simple exercises that can improve cardiovascular function and get everyone in better shape. Seek to work out at least twice a week, but not more than four days before you build up your endurance and strength.

Focus on perfecting your shape to get any workout completed correctly:

- Start with eight reps each (except where noted) for a set, and increase slowly by one or two reps each week. It will last for beginners 6 to 8 weeks, or even longer.

- If you're confident with 12 reps so you can hold the right shape, drop down to 8 reps but do two sets.

- Continue to add reps until 12 and continue with eight reps with three sets.

Another way to improve your workout is to add new exercises to the basics group gradually. With the 12 basics, several variations can be developed that work with various muscles and bring more of a challenge to your workout. 'Amping-up the Modern Workout' includes tips and guidance for more advanced versions of these basic muscle mass and strength-building exercises.

Remember, ALL workouts will start with a warm-up and finish with a cool down. This is important, but it's very easy as well. Just stretching and running in place for 2 to 3 minutes or anything similar is all it takes that can make the difference between a fantastic workout and a boring one.

Bridges

- Lay down your arms to the sides of your back, knees bent, and feet flat on the floor.
- Raising your butt and thighs off the floor while holding your abs close.

Burpees

- Stand straight with hip-width of feet apart.

- Keep an erect posture with your head in line with your spine, take a big step forward, and get your back heel off the floor.

- Lower the body to about 90 degrees for both knees to bend.

- Hold your abs close and take a diaphragm breath deep.

- Lift the front foot back, and return to standing.

- Bjujhr hSwap legs for one rep, and repeat.

Crunches

- Lie back with your legs on your side, one over the other. You can extend your lower arm to balance or bend in front of your body while the upper arm can rest on your side or over your waist.

- Lift your upper leg towards your shoulder and forward your shoulder, trying to put your ribs and hips together.

- Raise your leg for one rep and relax your shoulder.

- Switch to one set of sides to complete.

Chin touch

- Pull yourself so that your chin touches the bar from the dead hanging position with hands shoulder-width apart and palms facing off.
- Lower yourself, with leverage, for 6 to 8 reps.
- Don't kick or strike.

Pull-Ups

- Start building those muscles with flexed arm hangs if you can't perform a regular pull up.
- Use a stool or exercise buddy to get into the pull-up position, face above the bar, and hold that position as long as possible.

- For aggressive pull-ups, use a stool or exercise buddy to get into the chin-up position and lower yourself as slowly as possible.

These exercises work gravitationally and help you build muscle strength and grip—reverse hand grip (pronounced palms) for chin-ups.

Squatting

- Stand with spreading legs, feet slightly further apart than shoulder width. (Pointing your feet slightly outwards helps balance.)
- Bend your knees and sink your ass as if you were sitting on a chair.

- Down, so your thighs are parallel to the ground, then just go a little further – slightly below parallel.

- Maintain balance on the floor with feet flat and arms extended in front, if possible.

- Push your heels and straighten your legs to return to the starting position.

- Try to keep the body straight, leaning forward to maintain balance and execute the squat just as far as possible.

Oblique Leg Lifts

- Lie straight on your back, legs straight and arms slightly away from your sides, palms down. (Place a folded towel under your bottom back, just above your hips or bring your hands under your ass.)

- One choice is to bend your legs so that your knees are parallel to the floor.

- Then straighten your legs and gradually lower your feet to about 1 inch above the floor for one rep before bringing back your knees.

- The second option is to bend your legs and then extend them to the ceiling while pointing your toes before lowering the straight legs to just above the floor.

- Another option is to lift your legs straight from the ground without bending your knees, and then lower them straight.

- Repeat in a single package for a total of 5 reps. Holding the abs tight, breathing out as you lift your thighs, breathing in as you lower them, stop arching the back.

Planks

- Lie on your stomach, arms straight ahead.

- Raise your arms and legs off the floor with no joints closed.

- The aim is to create an arch with hips and shoulders off the floor.

- Hold for 3 to 5 seconds and get back to starting.

CHAPTER ELEVEN: ADDITIONAL EXERCISES IN CALISTHENICS

Arm Circles

- Standing apart (or sitting upright) with your feet shoulder-width, extend your arms' full length at shoulder height on the sides.

- Carry out small circular motions for 15 to 20 reps.

- Turn the circle over and continue for another 15 to 20 reps.

- Vary the scale or velocity of the circles to work different muscles in various angles.

Bend & Reach

- Start in a standing position, with feet slightly larger than the width of your shoulder apart and arms straight over your head.

- Squat, keeping feet flat and arms straight on the floor.

- Round the back as you squat, reaching out as far as possible between your thighs.

- Return to Start Position for a full rep.

Calf Raises

- Keep your feet close together. (Stand with your hands, if necessary)

- Raise the feet and stay for 5 seconds.

- Slowly lower your heel to the floor using leverage.

- Work on one foot at a time for flexibility, or stand on a step or stable platform to let your heels drop below your toes.

Tips

- Stand up against a solid bench, table, or low bar with your back. Add your hands to the side and stick your feet out in front of you.

- Lean slightly forward and lower your body, bend at the elbows until your elbow reaches an angle of around 90 degrees.

- Use the triceps muscles to lift yourself up to a full arm extension.

Free Hand and Neck Resistance– front, back, and side

- Stand with your feet comfortably apart, keeping the neck in a straight line.

- (Front) Press the head against your hands with your fingers interlocked and hands against your forehead.

- Start with the head back and push the resisting hands into your hands.

- (Back) Again, place your hands on the back of the head with your fingers interlocked.

- Start by pushing your head forward, back against your hands.

- (Side) Place your palm on the side of your head and resist as you move your head towards that direction.

- Switch to the opposite side and repeat.

Mountain Climbers

- Stand upright, or sit straight, lean your head forward and put your hands to your mouth.

- Roll your head to your right and try to touch your ear to your right shoulder.

- Tilt your head backward and raise your chin as high as possible.

- Tilt your head to your left and attempt to touch your ear to your left shoulder.

- Complete two full turns, rest for 30 seconds, then repeat in the opposite direction (left).

Prisoner Squats

- Stand straight, arms long, hands behind your back. You should have your elbows and shoulders back, and your heart braced.

- Bend your knees and bring your shoulders down and back.

- Keep your feet flat on the floor and put parallel thighs to the floor.

- Hold for a few seconds and use your thighs and hips to slowly raise yourself back up.

Russian Twists

- Sit down on the floor, knees bent, and feet on the floor together.

- Sit back at an angle of 45 degrees and gently move the shoulders from side to side, bending from the waist.

- The further from your body you hold your hands, the harder it'll be! Start with your hands crossed over your arms, then stretch tightly to your sides with your elbows in front. Finally, keep them loose in front of you.

- The more you twist, the more you reach core tightening.

- Take your feet off the floor to make your workout more intense.

Step-ups

- It's like walking up stairs except you're using just one.

- Stand up straight, step up on a sturdy platform, or step-up.

- Return the other foot to the floor after the total straightening of the knee.

- Complete the reps with one leg and then switch to the other.

Straight Leg Deadlift (Romanian)

- Stand with slightly separated feet.

- Lift your right leg up behind you as you bend straight back from the hips.

- Slightly bend your left knee to balance, and parallel your torso and leg to the floor.

- Return to standing position and move to full rep legs.

The Windmill

- Stand apart with feet slightly larger than the width of the shoulder and arms straight out of the shoulders, palms facing down.

- Continue turning from the waist to the left, holding arms in a straight line, and moving in line with the spine (not bent or turned).

- Bend your shoulders and raise your legs slightly as you reach forward to place your right hand on the outside of the left foot.

- Return to starting position and repeat one complete rep on the opposite leg.

Special note about the handstand!

Handstands are not necessarily considered exercises, but as advancing to handstand pushups is part of the overall

calisthenics and BWT plan, it is worth mentioning. To get the feeling of holding your body upright over your head, starting with a headstand may be easier.

- Get down on your knees in the push position

- Place your head between your elbows and your hands on the floor at 90 degrees

- Raise your bottom-up and balance your head and hand weight

- Place your hands on your elbows and raise your legs up into the air, one at a time.

Try the handstand once you get a feel for the balance. It could include a spotter who can help you lift your feet and assist you while you seek to maintain equilibrium.

- Lean forward as if you were doing a deadlift on one knee

- As you reach the ground with your hands push off on the ground with your foot

- Bring both feet together and bend your hands to strike a balance

This is likely to take quite a few attempts as you get the feeling of ending up yourself. It is the part where muscle regulation and the body's deliberate maneuvering around space plays a major role! Another way to learn how to perform a handstand is by using a prop, such as a wall or a tree.

- Press your feet against the prop from shortened push-up stance

- 'Walk' your feet up the prop as you walk closer to the prop

- Try removing both feet from the support when you're relatively upright and developing your balance

- Try to get into the stance from the upright, free-standing position as shown above once you have the power and balance to maintain the handstand.

CHAPTER TWELVE: APPLICATIONS OF CALISTHENICS TRAINING

The versatility of calisthenics and bodyweight training exercises encourage people of all ages, sizes, and physical conditions to have a plan. With so many potential exercises and endless combinations, the strength, endurance, and stability of beginners and professional athletes, as well as the disabled and rehabbing people, will benefit from cals and BWT. It is not difficult to work calisthenics and bodyweight exercise into any current program for people used to physical fitness activities. The beauty is that the results of this type of workout are so remarkable that you will be making it your primary training tool!

People who are just beginning should always work with their health care provider to determine how much to do and how easy to make progress. However, regardless of your situation, there

are plenty of exercises that will get you going to develop your endurance and the desire to do more.

WARMING UP AND GETTING STARTED

To that the risk of injury, everybody needs to do some warm-up exercises before exercising during an exercise program. A couple of minutes of cardio and some dynamic stretches will make a significant difference in your workout performance. On this practice, the body responds instinctively:

- Cardiovascular response: Blood flow is targeted to increase muscle function and heart rate, stroke volume, and systolic blood pressure.

- Circulatory responses: The improved blood flow makes it easier for the cells to eliminate toxins and also provides enough space for better cushioning of the joints.

- Respiratory responses: Respiratory muscles are designed to increase the ventilation rate and volume to improve lung and body tissue exchange.

- Musculoskeletal responses: Increases in body temperature due to increased blood flow. This helps lower muscle rigidity and increases the motion range.

- Nervous system responses: Neural pathways (throwing of the nerves from the brain to the muscles and back again) are activated to maintain smooth movement patterns.

- Metabolic responses: Hormone levels, particularly glucagon, are preparing to raise blood glucose levels for increased energy.

Taking into consideration the idea of CNS training, warm-ups should imitate the movements that you intend to perform during your workout. Before you send it, it is just like reading through a speech, so it runs seamlessly and does not pose any surprises. It also helps you to adjust the range of motion gently to prepare for the demands of your next routine or athletic event. Because of the value of heating, it is important to do it correctly. Such movements must be performed properly, just like using the appropriate stance and pose for any task, and not hurried or shortened. 2 to 3 minutes of warm-ups will be enough for basic workouts as long as you practice the muscle groups that will be used in your goal exercises. It requires up to 5 to 10 minutes of preparatory warm-ups for more intense or advanced exercises to ensure full body activation. Keep all aspects of the body in mind when doing warm-up stretches.

Arms

• Sit up straight apart from the foot of the neck.

• Elevate your right arm above your head and bend your elbow to the back of your head

• With left hand grip the elbow and pull softly, bending slightly to the left.

• Restrain for 15 – 20 seconds and relax, repeat 2 or 3 times, then turn sides.

Arms and Shoulders

• Sit up straight apart, steps wide of the neck.

- Extend your arms behind your back, your elbows straight, and your palms face each other (link your fingers if possible)

- Heat up arms slightly and keep for 15 to 20 seconds, then relax 2 to 3 times

Arms and Mid-Back

- Sit up straight apart, steps wide of the neck.

- Extend your arms straight in front of you, your elbows straight, and your palms face each other (link your fingers if possible)

- Move your hands forward without bending, to stretch your back.

- Store for 15 to 20 seconds, relax, repeat 2 to 3 times

Back, Core And Obliques

- Stand straight with feet larger than the width of your shoulder and arms straight to your sides, shoulder level.

- Gently twist your upper body to one side as far as possible, without leaning forward.

- Take 20 to 30 seconds and return to the forward position

- Repeat 2 or 3 times (or change sides for a minimum of 4 to 6 twists) and switch sides.

Calf and Quad Stretch

- Stand slightly spread over feet, about two feet apart and face the wall

- With feet flat on the floor and straight aft, lean towards the wall

- Calm and repeat for 15 to 20 seconds, 2 or 3 times

- Hold your right hand against the wall, then raise your right foot and grab it with your left hand behind you.

- Pull your foot gently back to the butt for 20 to 30 seconds, and then relax.

- Repeat two or three times, and switch sides

Thighs stretch

- Squat between your legs and place both hands on the floor

- Extend one leg straight behind you and keep the other foot flat on the floor

- Lean over your bent knee and hold for 20 to 30 seconds

- Turn your weight backward, your leg extended and hold for 20 to 30 seconds

- Relax and repeat and turn legs for 2 or 3 stretches

Hamstrings

Note that there are many stretching options for the hamstrings, and this is just one!

- Stand one foot straight ahead, a good foot-step length

- Bend your back straight from the hip and touch the floor on either side of your toes

- Save 20 to 30 seconds, relax, repeat 2 or 3 times and then turn sides

Static Warm-up loop stretches for hips and thighs.

Exercises that stretch double as a warm-up:

- Arms – forearms, biceps, and triceps – Circles of arms, Push up

- Back – top, middle and bottom – Superman, Bend and Reach

- Hips, abdominals and obliques-Windmill planks

- The legs – the calf, the thigh, the heart, the neck, the groin, the ankle.

- Neck and shoulders (traps) – Rolling neck, resistance to freehand neck

The cooldown, just as critical as the warm-up, gives the body an opportunity to remove cellular waste and lactic acid that builds up during exercise. Similar stretches as those for a warm-up and slow walking help bring back the breath to normal and prevent

muscle cramps from occurring by releasing the tension caused by intense contraction.

If you ever feel you need to skip warm-ups or cool down, skip the warm-up or shorten it. Since you warm up to avoid muscle strain, you don't have to worry about as much with cals and BWT as you would about weight lifting or other kinds of intense strength workouts. As part of the workout, you can do easier combinations of cals and BWT exercises and build up strength, but you still have to give your body a chance to return to 'normal' after some form of activity.

BEGINNER LEVEL WORKOUT PLAN

The most simple workout schedule involves the five big exercises (and don't forget to hot ups and cool downs!):

1. Dips

2. Lunges

3. Pull ups

4. Push ups

5. Squats

Start with a set number of each of those exercises, such as 5 or 8, depending on your fitness level. If that's too fast, start with ten and/or add some more things like

- Crunches

- The Windmill

- Calf Raises

Gradually add one or two reps per week until you double your starting number of reps. Drop back to that starting number again but do 2 complete sets each week, building up the number of reps. Take a brief break between sets (one or two minutes) to

catch your breath, but not long enough to refresh. Cut back on the rest in between, as you work easily with the number of reps in each set. Once you can comfortably do three sets, drop down the number of reps halfway to your original start number and add one exercise at a time from the list in Chapter 7, such as:

- Burpee

- Russian twists

- Bridges

- Superman

- Leg Lifts

- Mountain Climbers

- Step Ups

- Prisoner Squats

Be sure to pick a range of movements for a full-body workout, targeting specific muscle groups. Remember to keep the proper

shape and a tight core. If your technique fails, don't raise your reps! Doing a few exercises correctly is better than doing a lot of them wrong – you might be preventing real progress or even heading for injury!

TIMING YOUR WORKOUTS

A significant part of balancing your performance is scheduling your workouts. For beginners, doing calisthenics and exercises on body weight 2 or 3 times a week for 20 to 30 minutes is a good objective. This also depends on the workout's types of exercises. You have already been advised to select exercises that reach multiple muscle groups. Another factor is to balance fitness and energy, as well as choices in terms of impact and non-impact to avoid stress on the joints and muscles.

Swimming is a perfect choice, very gentle on the joints. Many of the cals and BWT can be done in the water that protects the joints and provides support whilst adding resistance. Older people and those in need of physical therapy can benefit greatly from exercising in the water, as well as being a great break for any athlete who needs to tone it down a little.

When you're in a consistent routine and improve with endurance and strength, you can increase your workouts to 4, 5, or even seven a week. Only bear in mind the scale, alternating days of mainly cardio with days of first and foremost strength exercises. (Many of the same exercises can actually be done for both purposes – quickly for cardio and slowly for strength!)

Another interesting choice is to do any type of activity that increases your heart rate in a few shorter periods as long as you reach a total of 30-60 minutes per day. This is perfect for busy

people because instead of using an elevator, rake leaves or mop a floor, carrying a child, a bag of groceries, or a laundry basket, you can climb stairs-you get the idea! Not only can you get a full workout in, but by firing it up more than once, you double the metabolic boost that you get and increase afterburn.

CREATE TIME FOR REST

While it is possible to do basic calisthenics and bodyweight exercises every day, it is important to remember the need for rest on the body. This is particularly true when you've engaged in more complex, higher intensity workouts that last until you experience 'the wall' or muscle failure. The muscles grow in mass and increase in strength, breaking down and rebuilding afterward. This rebuilding must have a chance to take place, so strength training workouts for those specific muscle groups

should have 24-48 hour breaks.

To be more precise, pulling ups, dips, and squats require a high degree of strength and greater muscle recruitment, particularly when you're doing a large number of reps and sets. To allow those muscles to rest and recover your cellular strength, they should not be done every day. Replace those workouts over alternate days with more stretches and cardio-based options.

Also, endurance training needs some rest, at least once a week, or at most every ten days. Take a slow stroll, doggy-paddle in a pool, or do some easy yoga if you can't just relax. This is healthy for both your mind and your body. It is also important that you get enough sleep every day, in addition to recovery from muscular efforts. Sleep deprivation accounts for a wide range of negative effects, the most important of which (in terms of weight loss and fitness) involves disruption of hormone

production (related to diabetes and Human Growth Hormone for muscle recovery and building) and also influence on the quality of the food choices we make.

INCREASE YOUR INTENSITY WITH PROGRESSIVE TRAINING

Calisthenics and exercises on bodyweight can help anybody build a better body. Although cals and BWT are ideally suited for stamina and lean muscle mass, it is also possible to achieve power and pumped up muscles by increasing cals and BWT workout speed. Similar workout positions target slightly different muscle groups.

- For pushups and pull-ups, keep the hands closer to the midline and further apart than the shoulder width to build depth and mass all around.

- Using leg heights and/or torso twist to pull up results in killer abs.

- Performing single-armed or single-legged pushups, squats, and other exercises double the strength.

- Requiring a greater balance leads to more muscle involvement.

This creates a strong body by having full control over your muscles and their work. Again, take a picture of a gymnast performing a routine, a ballet dancer, or an expert in martial arts: total concentration and a highly developed CNS link between the brain and muscles make movements that defy gravity all but. This only happens after a tremendous amount of repetition and

long hours of practice, during which the exercise's difficulty is steadily increased. Reps and sets are initially required to improve strength, flexibility, and endurance, but the real power and muscle building comes from more complex, fully functional movements that involve multiple joints and stabilizer muscles. This is where weight lifting differs so much from cals and BWT!

This is called 'Progressive Learning, ' which requires only the basic exercises with a variety of increasingly more challenging combinations. Changing the body's range of motion and leverage, along with overall positioning, provides the escalating challenge. Finally, from a move on your feet, you can push up to a handstand and even push up a one-armed handstand!

CHAPTER THIRTEEN: AMPLIFYING YOUR BASIC WORKOUT

By applying physics to physiology, anyone can turn a simple calisthenics and bodyweight training routine into an intense muscle-building session. What this means is that you can amp up your workout without using weights or any other equipment to build muscle and grow a great body by making some simple changes to your positioning. Just like a kid who has to crawl before he can walk, everybody who wants to make great progress with cals and BWT needs to start at the edge. Movement accuracy and attention to posture and shape are key elements of successful muscle building, so mastering the basics is critical for future improvement.

PRINCIPLES OF ADVANCED WORKOUTS

Relatively simple adjustments to your routine will significantly affect your overall performance. Looking at certain basic facts will add a great deal to your system as you learn the fundamentals and are ready to move on. This basic understanding of the difference between the concepts of fitness and weight lifting all around enables you to achieve practically every target you set in terms of strength and muscle mass by calisthenics and bodyweight training.

1. Work harder, not necessarily longer- The key to building muscle is to do less but more vigorous reps. The key to building muscle is to work towards fatigue, take a rest, and then work the same muscles in several sets again.

2. Isolate Key Muscles - Although cals and BWT ensure greater full-body strength, main muscle groups can be separated for big workouts. Focusing on one group of

muscles develops certain muscles more efficiently at a time.

3. Divide and conquer - It is easy to provide rest for a worked muscle group by dividing up your workouts according to item 2. Work on the shoulders and arms one day, then work on the legs the next. You should concentrate on the chest and back the third day, and then continue with the shoulders and arms the next day. You will practice every week for six days and then take a full day to heal overall.

4. Concentrate on functional movement - The beauty of cals and BWT is that many of the exercises imitate everyday activity. Make sure to capitalize on that and have moved in all three planes – side by side, front by back and rotating or twisting.

5. Keep the movement steady and regulated - Bouncing creates a kind of momentum, and you don't want it to make it easier to work out. Contract the muscles that you operate as hard as you can and keep the position for at least 5 seconds to maximize the time under stress. Limit rest periods to force the muscles to work harder, so that lactic acid has no chance to dissipate until your training session is complete.

6. To increase complexity, reduce leverage - The more your muscles are stretched out, the harder they have to work out to do an exercise. Pushups will start at shoulder width with your hands then raise the distance between your hands to be harder to operate. This definition involves adjusting the weight distribution and using

asymmetric positions (which lead to exercises with one arm and one leg).

7. Increase each motion 's length. This can be used for many movements, such as placing your feet on a block for pushups, squats, or lunges, using a higher platform for step-ups, and incorporating moves such as adding a hop to the basic toe-touch stand-up feature. Another way to get something out of each rep is to start the transfer but only return part-way to get going. You then return to the full-out role and usually return to get started. This can be performed once or as mini-reps to maximize total muscle activity within each rep.

8. Apply balance to any workout - By pushing the muscles to compensate for off-balance exercises, particularly the heart, you are through the overall work done. It can be done simply by shifting with one arm or one leg or by

going from a plank to a push-up or kneeling push-up to a push-up on the feet.

9. In one exercise, combine the plyometrics and isometrics- Add your stepping exercises with a jump or push off the floor during a pushup. Simply hop the muscles to fire for explosive strength and speed, and add to your aerobic workout.

10. Don't depend on elastic strength -Muscles are like coiled springs, such that the opposite movement normally accompanies each motion. By holding a position for at least 4 seconds, the natural recoil effect is reduced, so that the return motion depends entirely on the strength of the muscle.

11. Aim for progressive overloading. You have to constantly demand more from those muscles for the greatest muscle mass enhancements. Increase sets, the number of times

you work out every week, and the difficulty of the exercises you do (without compromising on good form). 'Convict conditioning,' also known as 'old school calisthenics,' is a common method to slowly increase the difficulty of exercises in optimizing intensity based on the experience and techniques of the fortified men, gymnasts, circus performers, and old acrobats.

12. To maximize your workout, perform supersets. A superset includes exercises that target completely different muscle groups so you can work with each group to near exhaustion, give them rest, and re-target them for what is called 'intensity training,' leading to 'cumulative fatigue.' You do a small number of reps but a lot of sets within 15 or 20 minutes of work.

CHAPTER FOURTEEN: HEART RATE BOOSTING EXERCISES

BURPEE

The burpee is the workout that so many of us love to hate, as it is one of the easiest ways to jack the sky-high heart rate.

REQUIREMENTS:

The typical burpee is performed by squatting down and positioning the shoulder width of your hands opposite you. From there, jump back into a board position on both of your feet and push up (see here). Jump your feet back to your hands at the top of the push-up, and stand up with enough energy to climb into the air with your hands reaching overhead. The real difficulty is not the number but the consistency of the reps. As

other calisthenics drills, there is a propensity for very high reps to do burpees, which can result in a lack of technical consistency. As I've advised with other exercises, the quality of your movements should be your priority, rather than the quantity or speed of your reps.

GOAL:

Aim to fill in 15 to 20 reps.

RESULTS:

If this is a point of struggle for you, you can omit the push-up, or you can bring your hands down to an elevated surface, like a weight bench, to make the exercise easier. If you are looking for more reward, aim to jump forward rather than straight up.

SKI HOPS

Ski hops are a basic jumping exercise I like to give to folks as they prepare for the ski season. Ski hops develop lower-body endurance in a way that mimics tearing down a bumpy ski slope.

REQUIREMENTS:

Choose a line or seam on the floor with your feet close together and your toes pointing slightly towards the line. Hop about one foot forward with both feet, land on the other side of the line, move your feet slightly, so your toes keep pointing toward the ground. Hop down the line without stopping or pausing for room length.

GOAL PERFORMANCE:

Try to move a distance of around 20 to 30 yards or 20 to 30 seconds each time your sets are.

Keep your knees bent, and stay on your feet balls. This will let you readily absorb the impact of each landing as well as leap into the next hop.

RESULTS:

The best way of varying this technique is to change the width and distance of your jumps. It's usually best to keep your hops fast and short, but if you need more of a challenge, feel free to stretch out your jumps to cover more ground.

CROSS-PUNCH WITH FRONT KICKS

This drill builds off the level 1 cross-punch exercise (see here), only now are you adding a kick between each set of punches with every leg. The kicks will make it harder for your legs than they do when you keep a static stance. This additional challenge will

not only increase the heart rate but will also require greater stability and coordination.

REQUIREMENTS:

Start this drill the same way you do cross-punches: with your feet far apart and your knees bent. Do a cross-punch with each arm, then move the entire weight to one side. In a front kick, send the other foot straight forward. Bend the knee and place it on the floor to draw the foot back in. Then move your weight to that leg and repeat on the other leg the same operation. Once you've got both legs back on the floor, do two more punches and repeat. Make sure you get back to a wide position after each blow, with both knees bent. This wider position will make you more comfortable and lower the tension on your knees, thus making the exercise more successful.

GOAL:

Try to complete 25 to 50 reps, where it counts as one rep to punch with each fist and to kick with each knee.

Don't be tempted to rush this exercise, as a lot of twisting forces are at work here. Instead, strive to keep movements smooth and transition steadily.

RESULTS:

As in the cross-punch exercise, adjust the height of your punches and kicks to give the practice a special coordinating challenge.

POWER UP WORKOUT

The basic model for this workout uses a mix of heart rate enhancing movements along with strength exercises to increase

the level of variation and coordination during the workout. Just modify this template to suit your fitness needs, as always.

TWO ROUNDS OF:

- LEG Lifts HAND 15 reps

- PLANKS AFTER 1 minute

- SKI 20-30 seconds

THREE ROUNDS OF:

8 Reps ARCHER PUSH-UPS by hand

12 Reps: PULL-UPS

HANDSTAND IN 5 reps

LEVERS OFF 10 seconds

Lower body and core training

TWO ROUNDS OF:

30 seconds per side STARFISH PLANKS

RAISES SINGLE-LEG CALF 20 reps per side

Cardio / strainbow

ROUND FOUR:

15 Reps to BURPEES

TOWEL HANGS 20 minutes

CROSS-PUNCH 1 minute WITH FRONT KICKS

CHAPTER FIFTEEN: RESTORATION AND FLEXIBILITY

A decent workout doesn't consist of pushing yourself as hard as possible. Only when you push your body to its limits does a workout not help. In fact, some of the most effective methods of training you can practice will actually help to reduce stress on your mind and body. Recovery exercises, like those in this chapter, offer you the opportunity to let your mind and body "downshift" from a sympathetic to a parasympathetic condition. This helps your body return to a more peaceful state where your heart rate is normal, and your mind is calm.

Cool Down stretches

Taking time to cool down after a long flight would be like landing an aircraft. Failure to follow methods of recovery is akin to sending the plane up into the atmosphere and then actually

letting it drop when it runs out of gas. While your cool-down exercises can be missed, doing them ensures you stay in charge, so you're less likely to crash later on. In our hectic modern lives, these techniques are particularly important, where we rarely take the time to relax and rejuvenate. Practicing these basic techniques will do wonders to relieve your physical and mental stress, which not only helps you heal from intense workouts but also from busy working days.

For each of the suggested cool-down stretches, the following recommendations apply:

Target:

Try to complete one to two sets, keeping each stretch per set for 20 to 30 seconds.

Stretching is supposed to be a form of exercise which is beneficial and not something you can force. Ease into each stretch until the targeted muscles feel a gentle tug. Keep the strip of light when respiring smoothly.

RESULTS:

Experiment with minor differences in placements in your hand and foot. Adjusting the height or width of your hands and feet can improve your stability and help you accentuate the muscles you are targeting.

STANDING QUAD STRETCH

The quad stretch at the front of the thighs and hips is one of the easiest ways to stretch out the muscles. This is an especially

useful way of releasing stiffness, which accumulates for long periods of time after sitting.

REQUIREMENTS:

Practice this stretch for stability and protection when keeping something like a tree or post sturdy on. Move your entire weight onto the leg nearest to your supporting side. Put your other foot up behind your hip by bending your knee as far as possible, bringing your foot toward your pelvis with your hand that doesn't hold onto your support. Starting there, move your bent leg knee gently backward until you feel a gentle stretch in the front of your body. Bring your knee forward after holding to release the stretch. Let go of your foot and turn your body to repeat on the other side to face the other direction.

Make sure you keep your body straight without bending forward or leaning back. Keeping your hips square is important; don't

twist or tilt your pelvis during the stretch. If you have trouble raising your foot up to your knees, you can place it behind you like a bench or chair on an elevated floor.

HANDS CLASP BEHIND STRETCH

This is one of my favorite movements to ease stress in your upper body and stretch out your shoulders front. This also encourages healthy posture and enhances breathing by "opening the mouth."

REQUIREMENTS:

Start by standing apart, with a tall stance, broad feet, and arm. Rise behind your back and clasp both hands' fingers together. Take a deep breath in and use your back muscles to pull down and back your arms as you bring the hands together. Hold the

stretch to relax before slowly letting go of your hands. A few times roll up your shoulders to shake off any tension in your upper body.

Depending on how you keep your hands behind your back, you can make this stretch easier or harder. Beginners might find that they need to grasp their fingertips or at first keep their hands quite open. You should be able to clasp your hands incomplete with your palms meeting over time. Push your palms together for the most advanced version without holding on to your hands at all, using only your back muscles to create the stretch.

SEATED TOE PULLS

The pressure on the seated toe extends virtually every muscle along the spine. It's also much more powerful than just leaning

over and trying to touch your feet because you're in control of the force rather than gravity.

REQUIREMENTS:

Start by sitting on the floor in front of you with your legs straight out. Bend your knees and move your hands forward, so you can hold your feet tightly on the balls. If you're wearing shoes, you might find it easier to get a grip. Straighten your legs gently until you feel a stretch of light in your hamstrings. When you're in, press your feet balls forward to stretch your back further. Make sure you breathe normally while holding this stretch. To relieve the stretch, pull your toes back and gently shake any stress around your hamstrings.

This is a very easy stretch to control since the further you push your feet out, the greater will be your stretch. On either your right hand to your left foot or vice versa, you can also aim to

reach diagonally across to get a twisting back and lat stretch.

SEATED TWIST

The seated twist can work wonders to relieve tension that may hide along your back, hips, and shoulders. It's also a perfect way to stretch tight muscles within your spine, which can be a source of headaches from stress.

REQUIREMENTS:

Start sitting on the floor in front of you with both legs straight out. Bend one knee and position it on the outside of the other leg (that stays flat on the ground). Twist your body to the bent knee and place the opposite arm on the outside of your leg. For stability, you might want to put the other hand behind you and

help hold your torso upright instead of letting it hunch over. Adjust your head and look in the direction you move as your breathing continues. Stop pressing your arm toward your knee to gently release the stretch. Repeat with the other hand. There are many ways this procedure can be modified, including changing how far you bend your knee or how much you twist. Do not push it to the point of pain for every run. Then keep a beam of light while taking deep breaths.

SIT-BACKS

This stretch is a perfect technique for loosening your lats while decompressing your spine as well. It simulates a hanging motion without requiring as much upper body strength and with easier means to adjust the intensity.

REQUIREMENTS:

Start the stretch that stands upright and holds onto a collection of suspension straps or a sturdy railing. Bend your knees and lean back with your hips, making a straight line between your hands and hips. Keep your weight on your feet flat, and breathe deeply as you let your ears lift up. Move the hips forward to stay out of the stretch and shake off some tension. If you use a suspension exercise, one side of your back can be accentuated by softly rotating your torso. If you use a stable bar, move your weight side by side to help stretch out one side and then the other side. The more weight you move, the longer the stretch is. Experiment with the versions of this stretch, both isometric and dynamic. Twist and hold in a smooth motion for a deep isometric stretch, or twist side by side to maximize blood flow and work the steadiness out of your muscles.

STANDING ARM PULL

The standing arm pull a perfect complement to the sit-back stretch, because it targets the shoulder and arm sides.

REQUIREMENTS:

Start the stretch by finding robust upright support such as a post or the edge of a wall. Stand slightly in front of the support and reach slightly below the shoulder level behind you to position the palm of your closest hand. Place the opposite foot of the arm on the post in front of you with your feet shoulder-width apart, using a reverse posture. Twist your torso gently away from the post and build a stretch in your neck, shoulder, and chest. Keep releasing the stretch, before gently twisting again. Turn feet to face the other side of repetition. The movement of the standing

arm — like several other stretches — requires you to add a bit of pressure to ease the move. It encourages voltage control and stability, but care must be taken not to push the stretch as far as possible. Only add enough friction to create a mild stretch without feeling like you are trying to pull your arm out of the socket on your hip.

STANDING OVERHEAD SIDE REACH

This stretch is a great example of the fact that simple is best, at times. This stretch is perfect in its simplicity as a step to relieve stress and tension after hours of sitting at a desk during the workday.

REQUIREMENTS:

The exercise is very basic; stand apart with your feet shoulder-width and back of your shoulders. Get up as high as you can with one arm, without straining your arm or shoulder. Allow your hips to shift a few inches so that you gently lean to the side with your lowered fingers reaching to the ground. At the same time, your raised hand softly extends upward, reaching in the direction you bend. That should create a stretch along your entire bodyside, especially along your back and obliques. Gently breathe. To release the stretch, move the hips back to neutral. On the other hand, repeat.

This stretch can be practiced in both isometric and dynamic fashions, just remember to move smoothly, so you don't pull or strain your muscles. This is supposed to be more of a relaxed stretch than an aerobic workout. When you pass above, it's also tempting to twist yourself to the left. Twisting isn't harmful, but

it can weaken the distance that you're trying to reach.

LYING FRONT STRETCH

This unique stretch works your body's rear side while stretching the forehead. It is also an efficient way of exercising to stretch the upper back, an ability that is sorely lacking in our sit-and-slouch culture.

REQUIREMENTS:

Start by lying on the floor with your arms bent down to put your hands close to your chest. Lift your head off the floor and look forward while tucking your shoulder blades back and forth from your hands. Press the palms gently into the floor to lift your chest and extend your back. Press up until either you feel a light stretch along your front side or you have reached the limit of

how far you can lift. Hold as deep as possible while respiring, then lower your torso gently back to the floor.

Tension the muscles in your posterior chain, including your hamstrings, glutes, and spinal erectors, when doing this stretch. This will help the stress flow through your entire body, rather than pooling at a sensitive spot. During this stretch, the most common pinch point is the lower back. If you feel stress building up in your back, lower your torso a few inches or until you feel no strain any longer.

RESTORATIVE POSES

These poses are meant to help wind down your muscles and the nervous system after intense workouts. This cool downtime is a crucial part of a successful workout and is often ignored. Our

busy lives find completing a workout all too enticing, and then hurry to finish the next thing on our to-do list. I am not suggesting that you finish your workout too abruptly. Your nervous system remains in sympathetic dominance when you finish your workout without winding down, which promotes the fight-or-flight instincts of your body — a stressful state to spend the rest of your day in. Practicing these poses at the end of your workout for just a few minutes helps move your system down into a parasympathetic state. These poses reduce stress and foster a more rapid recovery. They may not look like much, but in your overall health and well-being, they can have a big influence.

POSE OF THE INFANT

With good reason, the pose of the infant is a hallmark in restorative yoga. This positions your upper body in an elongated

posture that helps with breathing while relaxing your lower back and hips passively.

REQUIREMENTS:

Place in on your hands and knees for this pose. Place your feet and knees next to each other, and spread the width of your hands apart. Point your toes back, and on the instep, your feet can rest. If this is uncomfortable, to reduce pressure points, you can practice this stretch on a towel or mat. Sit your hips back on your feet while you keep your hands in place so that your arms stretch out before you. Exhale and let your spine round slightly when you do so. Hold the position, and keep breathing as deeply as possible. Push your hands gently towards your chest when you're done, and force yourself up to a seated kneeling position.

RESULTS:

You may want to spread your knees apart if you have trouble sitting back on your feet, so you can fall between your thighs. You can also provide additional help by putting a support under your thighs, like a yoga block.

DEEP BELLY RESPIRATION

Deep belly respiration is an efficient way to switch from a sympathetic dominant nervous system to a dominant parasympathetic system. Sadly, such deep breathing is becoming increasingly rare as our busy lifestyles leave us vulnerable to breathing shallowly in the lungs. Practicing this deep breathing method can do wonders for the overall stress levels after each

workout.

REQUIREMENTS:

Place your arms where they are most comfortable: on your hands, spread overhead, or extended out to the floor. Find a position that is totally comfortable, so you feel like you're melting into the floor. You can turn your head to either side, but I think it's best to put something soft under your forehead so that you can keep your neck neutral. Begin the breathing exercise once you're in place by inhaling as deep a breath as you can through your nose. When you breathe in, let your torso stretch through the floor in every direction, even to the sides, and even up and down to lengthen your spine slightly. Let your breath take off when you exhale in a relaxed way instead of blowing out violently. Go on for as many breaths as you like.

POSE OF THE LYING CHAIR

The pose of the lying chair is just like the pose of the lying front (see here), only now do you face the floor with your back and your knees bent to bring some height to your legs.

REQUIREMENTS:

You can do this either by folding your knees down on the floor with your feet or by putting your legs on a chair. Raising your legs increases lower body flexibility and decompresses your thighs, knees, and ankles. After a rough leg workout or long walk, it is an especially calming pose. Make sure you concentrate on drawing your breath as far into your abdomen as possible to relieve any tension in your core muscles that you might be

carrying. Hold the breath for a second before taking a relaxed exhalation. I find it helps to imagine a deflating balloon as your body relaxes while exhaling and releases any tension in your hands, feet, and face. Continue to breathe as long as you want. Rollover to one side when you're done, and gently get off the floor. Be careful not to get up too fast, which may make you feel dizzy.

• Hold for 3 – 5 seconds and return to the floor for one rep. (Flex your feet so that your weight rests for some additional pressure on your heels).

Burpees (Thrusts to Squat Jump)

- Stand up straight with engaged abs and the back of the neck.
- Lower your hands to the squat position in front of your feet;

- Hold your arms straight on your hands and move your legs back to the position of the chair.

- Slide back into the squat position and stand up to complete one rep.

Crumbs

- Lie flat on your back; knees bent at 90 degrees, feet flat on the ground.

- Place your hands lightly behind your head, hold your arms along your sides, or cross them over your chest.

- Engage the abs and exhale while lifting the shoulder blades off the floor.

- Do not close your jaw or pinch your ears. Look up at the stars, and shift your rib cage to your thighs.

Jumping Pockets

• Stand upright on your feet, with your arms loosely fall on your hands.

• Wake up inhaling, spreading your feet, and knocking down your head.

• Spring up again in constant motion to get your feet back to the start and your arms back on your hands.

• Holding the abs close, and straight back.

• Make 20 to 30 reps for a set, maintaining a good pace.

SIT-CHAIR POSE

This stretch is a perfect technique for loosening your lats while decompressing your spine as well. It simulates a hanging motion

without requiring as much upper body strength and with easier means to adjust the intensity.

REQUIREMENTS:

Start the stretch that stands upright and holds onto a collection of suspension straps or a sturdy railing. Bend your knees and lean back with your hips, making a straight line between your hands and hips. Keep your weight on your feet flat, and breathe deeply as you let your ears lift up. Move the hips forward to stay out of the stretch and shake off some tension.

If you use a suspension exercise, one side of your back can be accentuated by softly rotating your torso. If you use a stable bar, move your weight side by side to help stretch out one side and then the other side. The more weight you move, the longer the

stretch is. Experiment with the versions of this stretch, both isometric and dynamic. Twist and hold in a smooth motion for a deep isometric stretch, or twist side by side to maximize blood flow and work the steadiness out of your muscles.

STANDING ARM PULL

The standing arm pulls a perfect complement to the sit-back stretch because it targets the shoulder and arm sides.

REQUIREMENTS:

Start the stretch by finding robust upright support such as a post or the edge of a wall. Stand slightly in front of the support and reach slightly below the shoulder level behind you to position the palm of your closest hand. Place the opposite foot of the arm on the post in front of you with your feet shoulder-width apart,

using a reverse posture. Twist your torso gently away from the post and build a stretch in your neck, shoulder, and chest. Keep releasing the stretch, before gently twisting again. Turn feet to face the other side of repetition.

The movement of the standing arm — like several other stretches — requires you to add a bit of pressure to ease the move. It encourages voltage control and stability, but care must be taken not to push the stretch as far as possible. Only add enough friction to create a mild stretch without feeling like you are trying to pull your arm out of the socket on your hip.

CHAPTER SIXTEEN: MINDSET AND NURTURING HEALTHY HABITS

In this chapter, the exercises are a great reminder that fitness isn't always about stressing you out. Many of the healthiest practices you can develop, include, eliminating tension from your mind and body instead of going around the other direction.

Yes, preparation can be a real challenge, and there will certainly be moments when you can force yourself beyond your comfort zone. Such occasions, however, should be more the exception than the norm. Acute, short-term stress moments can spur improvement. Chronic mental and physical stress, on the other hand, will suppress the stimulation and keep the body from improving much at all. I recommend adjusting how you do your workouts to avoid overpowering yourself and keep your training healthy for both mind and body. Every workout you don't have

to use a different routine, but play around with some of the variations that I have described for each technique. It is also vital that exercise is not treated as a form of punishment. With exercises that often leave you feeling tired and drained, you can not force yourself into shape. After each workout, some experts recommend "leaving a little in the tank," and I fully endorse that idea.

That also applies to mind training. No one in life ever achieved more by continuously berating with negative self-talk. If something, then the situation is the reverse. A genuinely effective exercise approach requires more than hard work and effort at the gym. This is another dimension of self-care and healing that is just as important as you perform the individual exercises.

In this chapter, I will discuss some of the key points that will

complement your physical fitness, including tips for safe self-care strategies and advice with a review of a positive workout log to create your own workout schedule. Recall that the self-care aspects discussed in this chapter are among the most frequently neglected aspects of a successful workout plan. You can accelerate your results by paying attention to these topics, while also making your training much more enjoyable.

REST AND SELF-WARNING

Stress is like medicine when you're fit. Stress improves wellbeing and development in the proper dosages. If you get the dose wrong, however, stress can poison both your body and mind and break your results rather than make them up. That's why the following tips are so important; they will help you to ensure that your training stress will stimulate the changes you want, rather

than preventing them from happening.

Sleep is the first significant part of wellbeing and recuperation. During your workouts, your body doesn't change; it changes — grows stronger, more flexible, and fitter — in recovery. And if you barely rest, the performance will be seriously compromised. Sleep is the main resting part. It is so important that I often tell people that improving their sleeping habits can be more beneficial to their goals of fitness than improving their combined diet and exercise program. Getting the best sleep will also be as high a priority as trying to stick to your diet and practice habits. I hope having enough sleep will help if you're struggling to make progress and run on little rest.

Aside from sleep, it is also important to rest from one particular activity. Working all out every day in your workouts delays recovery, allowing your muscles to relax a bit after your workouts

are necessary for building muscle and power. After highly fatigued workouts, a healthy, varied program will let the different muscle groups relax. There is also mental and emotional relief in healing. Meditation, relaxation and just plain fun isn't luxury. These are important in your wellbeing and should be followed daily. Give yourself time to blow off steam and do something that feels good. Sing and dance to your favorite music while driving away from work. During your lunch break, take a stroll along the nearby nature trail or in the woods. Speak to a friend about something else but work.

Pain management is another significant thing to remember when we talk of rest and healing as part of a good, safe lifestyle. The two main forms of pain are both internal and external pain. Superficial pain, including wounds, burns, and blisters, is skin deep. The most common superficial injuries in calisthenics are to

the hands and feet. These injuries can often be avoided or addressed with properly fitting apparel or gloves. If you live in a dry environment, you can find that applying a daily moisturizer will help avoid cracked skin. Skin softener helps a lot with the callous, which tends to build up through the practice of calisthenics, particularly with pulling techniques. In order to give your hands time to recover, it's best to avoid any textures or grips that aggravate an existing injury. As you build a regular practice of calisthenics, your skin will become tougher over time, helping to prevent further superficial injuries.

Internal pain is a much more serious problem and often occurs in the joints, ligaments, and tendons. Typically, tendon pain can be identified in the form of a sharp and burning sensation around a joint, especially when the joint is under a load. Tendon pain frequently occurs in joints with little muscular support such as

knees, elbows, and wrists. Pain should always be treated in these areas and should never be "worked over" or ignored. Doing so only leads to a greater degree of internal damage, which will often require more serious action in the future to address it.

Perhaps a sudden ache in a joint is merely an adjustment where something jiggles during the workout instead of zagging. In these cases, after a week or two of rest and light activity, the issue will go away to facilitate blood flow into the region. The application of heat can also increase blood flow and healing help. When pain lasts more than a few weeks, it is usually a sign that there is a misalignment or imbalance that causes tension to build up to where it shouldn't be. In this case, it is better to get the condition assessed by a professional — an athletic trainer, doctor, or physical therapist — who can diagnose the injury and allow it to be handled. Quite frequently, the movement you do

when you feel the discomfort is not causing the problem; it is showing it instead. So avoiding the painful technique may provide temporary relief but does not resolve the underlying problem, which has the potential to worsen over time.

The most important thing to consider is that what you hear will boost your healthy habits. They 're supposed to make you feel happy, more inspired, more energized, and minimize pain. If you start experiencing chronic fatigue, pain, or a general loss of motivation, there is a good chance that something will affect your mind and body detrimentally and should be addressed as soon as possible.

DEALING AND FRUSTRATION With SELF-DOUBT

The greatest threats to the success of your training are not

physical but rather mental and emotional. Mental challenges can also be more prejudicial to the goals than just a physical injury. Few things like self-doubt will hold you off. A lack of faith in your ability to succeed, while tempting you to look for reasons to quit, can drain you from motivation. The self-doubt is a natural part of any phase of development. Every time you try to improve your life, you venture into uncharted waters, and there is no telling what you may encounter along the way. It is completely natural to feel confused about what you are doing or what will happen. Actually, that's a very positive indication you 're pushing yourself and widening your horizons.

Frustration, on the other side of self-doubt. While self-doubt is preventing you from taking action, frustration comes after you take action, and the results are disappointed. The best way to do this is to use your frustration as a springboard to propel you.

Take stock of just how far you have come and realized that just making a little progress is 100% better than no progress at all. You may also recognize areas that you do not tackle, such as sleep, diet, or training, to see if there are any basic aspects that you can push forward.

Motivation is as important as the amount of physical strength. Ebbing and flowing along with life with highs and lows is natural for it. Sometimes during a couple of days, you may have low motivation. Other times, you may have weeks or even months of low motivation at a time. The good news is, while motivation can — and will — leave you, it will come back as well. That's why it's important to continue your training habits, even in times when motivation is beginning to wane. You will lose a lot of ground if you quit or take a long break, and you will be forced to make it all up when the next wave of motivation

comes in. When you no longer have the time or motivation to push as hard as you can, it's okay to scale back into your habits. Reduce the volume of your training or loosen your diet up a little. You don't have to stay perfect or do everything "right" all the time to keep progressing. You just have to carry on doing what you can, so you can ramp up later.

CREATE YOUR OWN WORKOUT PROGRAM

It can seem like a daunting task to create your own workout program, especially when you start out. Don't be afraid, my friend. One of the best things to start out is that this is the easiest time you can make progress in your training career. Hold in mind the following points, and you are going to be ready to go.

The first thing you need to do is to set your goals clearly, so you can develop your training plan accordingly. If you need a reminder about how to set your goals, and what eating and exercise habits will move you in the right direction, refer back to the material in the first chapter. Also, if you want to lose fat, you 're going to make your primary target burning calories. If muscle building is your goal, you'll want to challenge your muscles' strength and work capacity. And if your goal is a functional skill, you'll want to make sure your training challenges the specific functional capabilities you want to improve.

The next move is to prepare a typical week of workouts. Write your exercise schedule to a calendar that will last a week. I recommend starting with three full-body calisthenics workouts per week, for simplicity. Schedule the workouts on non-consecutive days such as Monday, Tuesday, and Friday. This

simple framework is useful for almost any target and has a long history of helping a number of individuals, from professional athletes to weekend warriors and senior citizens, achieve success.

The final step, once you've built a week-long schedule that's going to work for you, is to decide which exercises you'll include in each workout that week. Consider starting with the workout recipes I've given you for each of the three workout rates in the case of your Calisthenics training. Practice at least a few weeks of the Start Strong routine, and step up as you feel ready.

In the beginning, the most important thing is to get used to working and create continuity. In addition, concentrate on ensuring that your workouts guide you towards your goals. If your goal is to burn fat, your schedule will involve some form of physical activity most days of the week to increase burnt calories. Through training in calisthenics, you will definitely burn fat, but

you will also want to substitute with other exercises of your choosing to keep moving and burning. When the target you set is to create muscle, your bases will be covered by a three-day week schedule, and you'll want to rest in the other days to heal. In this case, focus on testing your muscles with each of your workouts very hard, usually with two or four sets of five to 20 reps.

Finally, if you're trying to develop a practical skill, your strength training schedule for three days a week should support your regular skill practice, whether it's hitting a golf ball or throwing a side-kick. Don't put any burden on your overall routine. Your routine should provide a sufficient framework to allow you to be deliberate and reflective in achieving your goals but not so rigid that it does not fit with your life. The main key ingredient for

your performance is not the routine's nitty-gritty — it's aligned with your fitness schedule, and you're getting better from one workout to another.

YOUR WORKOUT LOGBOOK

The success in the workout does not come from the workouts you are performing or the routine you perform. It comes from advancing the exercises that you are doing and the routine you practice. Keeping a fitness log is one of the most effective ways to ensure you are making progress. It's pretty easy to keep a log; just write down what you've done and any information on how you've done it. I suggest you find a format that would be convenient for you. Many people tend to keep their newspaper in a flat, lined notebook while others tend to use a computerized tablet. Personally, I use my mobile with a basic notepad feature,

and I always have it with me.

Discuss what you should do in the next exercise to advance the preparation after you have taken note of what you have done. Including doing a few reps to enhancing the technique, it can be something. Jotting down these notes and reflections gives you a set of directions for what to do in your next workout in order to continue moving forward towards your objectives.

Enjoy Your New Journey!!!

CONCLUSION

Congratulations on finishing this book, my friend! This may be a summary, but your career in calisthenics is just beginning. There are plenty of possibilities and resources to explore for you, and I'm still here to support you on your journey. Please bear in mind a few things as you begin your study. Firstly, exercise and physical fitness are designed to help you feel good and enhance the quality of your life. If you ever feel your wellbeing and life satisfaction eroding, stop and rethink your approach, please. Fitness habits that are neither healthy nor productive to compromise your well-being.

Firstly, listen to your body and confide in your instincts. Diet and exercise are far from being an absolute science; not all the solutions are open to even the leading experts. If you thought it would be a smart idea to make a change of strategy, then it is

worth acting on the feeling. Eventually, know you're going to

learn a lot more from personal experience than from any book.

Tools like this are great places to get ideas, but significant action

is the true source of information and understanding. Create the

strategy and take the first step. Wherever you go from here, is up

to you, and I'm sure it's going to be a fun lifelong journey that

will be satisfying.

CONTENTS

	Acknowledgments	i
1	Chapter Name	1
2	Chapter Name	Pg #
3	Chapter Name	Pg #
4	Chapter Name	Pg #
5	Chapter Name	Pg #
6	Chapter Name	Pg #
7	Chapter Name	Pg #
8	Chapter Name	Pg #
9	Chapter Name	Pg #
10	Chapter Name	Pg #

ACKNOWLEDGMENTS

Insert acknowledgments text here. Insert acknowledgments text here. Insert acknowledgments text here. Insert acknowledgments text here. Insert acknowledgments text here. Insert acknowledgments text here. Insert acknowledgments text here. Insert acknowledgments text here. Insert acknowledgments text here. Insert acknowledgments text here.

1 CHAPTER NAME

Insert chapter one text here. Insert chapter one text here. Insert chapter one text here. Insert chapter one text here. Insert chapter one text here. Insert chapter one text here. Insert chapter one text here. Insert chapter one text here. Insert chapter one text here. Insert chapter one text here. Insert chapter one text here.
Insert chapter one text here. Insert chapter one text here. Insert chapter one text here. Insert chapter one text here.

Insert chapter one text here. Insert chapter one text here. Insert chapter one text here. Insert chapter one text here. Insert chapter one text here. Insert chapter one text here. Insert chapter one text here. Insert chapter one text here. Insert chapter one text here. Insert chapter one text here.

Insert chapter one text here. Insert chapter one text here. Insert chapter one text here.

Insert chapter one text here. Insert chapter one text here. Insert chapter one text here. Insert chapter one text here. Insert chapter one text here. Insert chapter one text here. Insert chapter one text here. Insert chapter one text here. Insert chapter one text here. Insert chapter one text here. Insert chapter one text here.

Insert chapter one text here. Insert chapter one text here. Insert chapter one text here. Insert chapter one text here.

Insert chapter one text here. Insert chapter one text here. Insert chapter one text here. Insert chapter one text here. Insert chapter one text here. Insert chapter one text here. Insert chapter one text here. Insert chapter one text here. Insert chapter one text here.

Insert chapter one text here. Insert chapter one text here. Insert chapter one text here.

Insert chapter one text here. Insert chapter one text here. Insert chapter one text here. Insert chapter one text here. Insert chapter one text here.

Insert chapter one text here. Insert chapter one text here. Insert chapter one text here. Insert chapter one text here. Insert chapter one text here. Insert chapter one text here.

Insert chapter one text here. Insert chapter one text here. Insert chapter one text here. Insert chapter one text here.

Insert chapter one text here. Insert chapter one text here. Insert chapter one text here. Insert chapter one text here. Insert chapter one text here. Insert chapter one text here. Insert chapter one text here. Insert chapter one text here. Insert chapter one text here.

Insert chapter one text here. Insert chapter one text here. Insert chapter one text here. Insert chapter one text here. Insert chapter one text here. Insert chapter one text here. Insert chapter one text here. Insert chapter one text here. Insert chapter one text here. Insert chapter one text here. Insert chapter one text here. Insert chapter one text here. Insert chapter one text here. Insert chapter one text here.

Insert chapter one text here. Insert chapter one text here. Insert chapter one text here. Insert chapter one text here. Insert chapter one text here. Insert chapter one text here. Insert chapter one text here. Insert chapter one text here. Insert chapter one text here. Insert chapter one text here. Insert chapter one text here. Insert chapter one text here. Insert chapter one text here. Insert chapter one text here. Insert chapter one text here. Insert chapter one text here. Insert chapter one text here. Insert chapter one text here.

Insert chapter one text here. Insert chapter one text here. Insert chapter one text here. Insert chapter one text here.

Insert chapter one text here. Insert chapter one text here. Insert chapter one text here. Insert chapter one text here. Insert chapter one text here. Insert chapter one text here. Insert chapter one text here. Insert chapter one text here. Insert chapter one text here.

Insert chapter one text here. Insert chapter one text here. Insert chapter one text here. Insert chapter one text here. Insert chapter one text here. Insert chapter one text here. Insert chapter one text here. Insert chapter one text here. Insert chapter one text here. Insert chapter one text here.

Insert chapter one text here. Insert chapter one text here. Insert chapter one text here. Insert chapter one text here.

Insert chapter one text here. Insert chapter one text here. Insert chapter one text here. Insert chapter one text here. Insert chapter one text here. Insert chapter one text here. Insert chapter one text here. Insert chapter one text here. Insert chapter one text here.

Insert chapter one text here. Insert chapter one text here. Insert chapter

one text here. Insert chapter one text here. Insert chapter one text here. Insert chapter one text here. Insert chapter one text here. Insert chapter one text here. Insert chapter one text here. Insert chapter one text here. Insert chapter one text here.

Insert chapter one text here. Insert chapter one text here. Insert chapter one text here. Insert chapter one text here. Insert chapter one text here. Insert chapter one text here. Insert chapter one text here. Insert chapter one text here. Insert chapter one text here. Insert chapter one text here. Insert chapter one text here. Insert chapter one text here. Insert chapter one text here. Insert chapter one text here.

Insert chapter one text here. Insert chapter one text here. Insert chapter one text here. Insert chapter one text here. Insert chapter one text here. Insert chapter one text here. Insert chapter one text here. Insert chapter one text here. Insert chapter one text here. Insert chapter one text here. Insert chapter one text here.

2 CHAPTER NAME

Insert chapter two text here. Insert chapter two text here. Insert chapter two text here. Insert chapter two text here. Insert chapter two text here. Insert chapter two text here. Insert chapter two text here. Insert chapter two text here. Insert chapter two text here. Insert chapter two text here. Insert chapter two text here. Insert chapter two text here. Insert chapter two text here.

Insert chapter two text here. Insert chapter two text here.

Insert chapter two text here. Insert chapter two text here. Insert chapter two text here. Insert chapter two text here. Insert chapter two text here. Insert chapter two text here. Insert chapter two text here. Insert chapter two text here. Insert chapter two text here. Insert chapter two text here. Insert chapter two text here. Insert chapter two text here. Insert chapter two text here. Insert chapter two text here. Insert chapter two text here. Insert chapter two text here. Insert chapter two text here. Insert chapter two text here.

Insert chapter two text here. Insert chapter two text here. Insert chapter two text here. Insert chapter two text here. Insert chapter two text here. Insert chapter two text here. Insert chapter two text here. Insert chapter two text here. Insert chapter two text here. Insert chapter two text here. Insert chapter two text here. Insert chapter two text here. Insert chapter two text here. Insert chapter two text here. Insert chapter two text here. Insert chapter two text here. Insert chapter two text here. Insert chapter two text here.

Insert chapter two text here. Insert chapter two text here. Insert chapter two text here. Insert chapter two text here. Insert chapter two text here. Insert chapter two text here. Insert chapter two text here. Insert chapter two text here. Insert chapter two text here. Insert chapter two text here. Insert chapter two text here.

Insert chapter two text here. Insert chapter two text here. Insert chapter two text here. Insert chapter two text here. Insert chapter two text here. Insert chapter two text here. Insert chapter two text here. Insert chapter two text here. Insert chapter two text here. Insert chapter two text here. Insert chapter two text here. Insert chapter two text here. Insert chapter two text here. Insert chapter two text here.

Insert chapter two text here. Insert chapter two text here. Insert chapter two text here. Insert chapter two text here. Insert chapter two text here. Insert chapter two text here. Insert chapter two text here. Insert chapter two text here. Insert chapter two text here. Insert chapter two text here. Insert chapter two text here. Insert chapter two text here. Insert chapter two text here. Insert chapter two text here. Insert chapter two text here. Insert chapter two text here. Insert chapter two text here. Insert chapter two text here. Insert chapter two text here.

Insert chapter two text here. Insert chapter two text here. Insert chapter two text here. Insert chapter two text here. Insert chapter two text here. Insert chapter two text here. Insert chapter two text here. Insert chapter two text here. Insert chapter two text here. Insert chapter two text here. Insert chapter two text here. Insert chapter two text here. Insert chapter two text here. Insert chapter two text here. Insert chapter two text here. Insert chapter two text here. Insert chapter two text here. Insert chapter two text here.

3 CHAPTER NAME

Insert chapter three text here. Insert chapter three text here. Insert chapter three text here. Insert chapter three text here. Insert chapter three text here. Insert chapter three text here. Insert chapter three text here. Insert chapter three text here. Insert chapter three text here. Insert chapter three text here. Insert chapter three text here. Insert chapter three text here.

Insert chapter three text here. Insert chapter three text here. Insert chapter three text here. Insert chapter three text here. Insert chapter three text here. Insert chapter three text here. Insert chapter three text here. Insert chapter three text here. Insert chapter three text here. Insert chapter three text here. Insert chapter three text here. Insert chapter three text here.

Insert chapter three text here. Insert chapter three text here.

Insert chapter three text here. Insert chapter three text here. Insert chapter three text here. Insert chapter three text here. Insert chapter three text here. Insert chapter three text here. Insert chapter three text here.

Insert chapter three text here. Insert chapter three text here.

Insert chapter three text here. Insert chapter three text here.

Insert chapter three text here. Insert chapter three text here.

Insert chapter three text here. Insert chapter three text here. Insert

chapter three text here. Insert chapter three text here.

4 CHAPTER NAME

Insert chapter four text here. Insert chapter four text here. Insert chapter four text here. Insert chapter four text here. Insert chapter four text here. Insert chapter four text here. Insert chapter four text here. Insert chapter four text here. Insert chapter four text here. Insert chapter four text here. Insert chapter four text here. Insert chapter four text here.

Insert chapter four text here. Insert chapter four text here. Insert chapter four text here. Insert chapter four text here. Insert chapter four text here. Insert chapter four text here. Insert chapter four text here. Insert chapter four text here. Insert chapter four text here. Insert chapter four text here. Insert chapter four text here. Insert chapter four text here.

Insert chapter four text here. Insert chapter four text here.

Insert chapter four text here. Insert chapter four text here. Insert chapter four text here. Insert chapter four text here. Insert chapter four text here. Insert chapter four text here. Insert chapter four text here. Insert

chapter four text here. Insert chapter four text here.

Insert chapter four text here. Insert chapter four text here.

Insert chapter four text here. Insert chapter four text here.

Insert chapter four text here. Insert chapter four text here. Insert

chapter four text here. Insert chapter four text here.

Insert chapter four text here. Insert chapter four text here.

5 CHAPTER NAME

Insert chapter five text here. Insert chapter five text here. Insert chapter five text here. Insert chapter five text here. Insert chapter five text here. Insert chapter five text here. Insert chapter five text here. Insert chapter five text here. Insert chapter five text here. Insert chapter five text here. Insert chapter five text here. Insert chapter five text here.

Insert chapter five text here. Insert chapter five text here. Insert chapter five text here. Insert chapter five text here. Insert chapter five text here. Insert chapter five text here. Insert chapter five text here. Insert chapter five text here. Insert chapter five text here. Insert chapter five text here. Insert chapter five text here. Insert chapter five text here.

Insert chapter five text here. Insert chapter five text here.

Insert chapter five text here. Insert chapter five text here. Insert chapter five text here. Insert chapter five text here. Insert chapter five text here. Insert chapter five text here. Insert chapter five text here. Insert chapter

five text here. Insert chapter five text here.

Insert chapter five text here. Insert chapter five text here.

Insert chapter five text here. Insert chapter five text here.

Insert chapter five text here. Insert chapter five text here. Insert chapter

five text here. Insert chapter five text here.

Insert chapter five text here. Insert chapter five text here.

6 CHAPTER NAME

Insert chapter six text here. Insert chapter six text here. Insert chapter six text here. Insert chapter six text here. Insert chapter six text here. Insert chapter six text here. Insert chapter six text here. Insert chapter six text here. Insert chapter six text here. Insert chapter six text here. Insert chapter six text here. Insert chapter six text here.

Insert chapter six text here. Insert chapter six text here. Insert chapter six text here. Insert chapter six text here. Insert chapter six text here. Insert chapter six text here. Insert chapter six text here. Insert chapter six text here. Insert chapter six text here. Insert chapter six text here. Insert chapter six text here. Insert chapter six text here.

Insert chapter six text here. Insert chapter six text here.

Insert chapter six text here. Insert chapter six text here. Insert chapter six text here. Insert chapter six text here. Insert chapter six text here. Insert chapter six text here. Insert chapter six text here. Insert chapter six text here. Insert chapter six text here. Insert chapter six text here. Insert chapter

six text here. Insert chapter six text here.

Insert chapter six text here. Insert chapter six text here.

Insert chapter six text here. Insert chapter six text here.

Insert chapter six text here. Insert chapter six text here. Insert chapter six text here. Insert chapter six text here. Insert chapter six text here. Insert chapter six text here. Insert chapter six text here. Insert chapter six text here. Insert chapter six text here. Insert chapter six text here. Insert chapter six text here. Insert chapter six text here. Insert chapter six text here. Insert chapter six text here. Insert chapter six text here. Insert chapter six text here. Insert chapter six text here. Insert chapter six text here. Insert

chapter six text here. Insert chapter six text here.

Insert chapter six text here. Insert chapter six text here.

7 CHAPTER NAME

Insert chapter seven text here. Insert chapter seven text here. Insert chapter seven text here. Insert chapter seven text here. Insert chapter seven text here. Insert chapter seven text here. Insert chapter seven text here. Insert chapter seven text here. Insert chapter seven text here. Insert chapter seven text here. Insert chapter seven text here. Insert chapter seven text here.

Insert chapter seven text here. Insert chapter seven text here. Insert chapter seven text here. Insert chapter seven text here. Insert chapter seven text here. Insert chapter seven text here. Insert chapter seven text here. Insert chapter seven text here. Insert chapter seven text here. Insert chapter seven text here. Insert chapter seven text here. Insert chapter seven text here.

Insert chapter seven text here. Insert chapter seven text here.

Insert chapter seven text here. Insert chapter seven text here. Insert

chapter seven text here. Insert chapter seven text here.

Insert chapter seven text here. Insert chapter seven text here.

Insert chapter seven text here. Insert chapter seven

text here. Insert chapter seven text here. Insert chapter seven text here. Insert chapter seven text here. Insert chapter seven text here. Insert chapter seven text here. Insert chapter seven text here. Insert chapter seven text here.

Insert chapter seven text here. Insert chapter seven text here.

Insert chapter seven text here. Insert chapter seven text here.

8 CHAPTER NAME

Insert chapter eight text here. Insert chapter eight text here. Insert chapter eight text here. Insert chapter eight text here. Insert chapter eight text here. Insert chapter eight text here. Insert chapter eight text here. Insert chapter eight text here. Insert chapter eight text here. Insert chapter eight text here. Insert chapter eight text here. Insert chapter eight text here.

Insert chapter eight text here. Insert chapter eight text here. Insert chapter eight text here. Insert chapter eight text here. Insert chapter eight text here. Insert chapter eight text here. Insert chapter eight text here. Insert chapter eight text here. Insert chapter eight text here. Insert chapter eight text here. Insert chapter eight text here. Insert chapter eight text here. Insert chapter eight text here.

Insert chapter eight text here. Insert chapter eight text here.

Insert chapter eight text here. Insert chapter eight text here. Insert chapter eight text here. Insert chapter eight text here. Insert chapter eight text here. Insert chapter eight text here. Insert chapter eight text here. Insert

chapter eight text here. Insert chapter eight text here.

Insert chapter eight text here. Insert chapter eight text here.

Insert chapter eight text here. Insert chapter eight text here.

Insert chapter eight text here. Insert chapter eight text here. Insert

chapter eight text here. Insert chapter eight text here.

Insert chapter eight text here. Insert chapter eight text here.

9 CHAPTER NAME

Insert chapter nine text here. Insert chapter nine text here. Insert chapter nine text here. Insert chapter nine text here. Insert chapter nine text here. Insert chapter nine text here. Insert chapter nine text here. Insert chapter nine text here. Insert chapter nine text here. Insert chapter nine text here. Insert chapter nine text here. Insert chapter nine text here.

Insert chapter nine text here. Insert chapter nine text here. Insert chapter nine text here. Insert chapter nine text here. Insert chapter nine text here. Insert chapter nine text here. Insert chapter nine text here. Insert chapter nine text here. Insert chapter nine text here. Insert chapter nine text here. Insert chapter nine text here. Insert chapter nine text here.

Insert chapter nine text here. Insert chapter nine text here.

Insert chapter nine text here. Insert chapter nine text here. Insert chapter nine text here. Insert chapter nine text here. Insert chapter nine text here. Insert chapter nine text here. Insert chapter nine text here. Insert

chapter nine text here. Insert chapter nine text here.

Insert chapter nine text here. Insert chapter nine text here.

Insert chapter nine text here. Insert chapter nine text here.

Insert chapter nine text here. Insert chapter nine text here. Insert

chapter nine text here. Insert chapter nine text here.

Insert chapter nine text here. Insert chapter nine text here.

10 CHAPTER NAME

Insert chapter ten text here. Insert chapter ten text here. Insert chapter ten text here. Insert chapter ten text here. Insert chapter ten text here. Insert chapter ten text here. Insert chapter ten text here. Insert chapter ten text here. Insert chapter ten text here. Insert chapter ten text here. Insert chapter ten text here.

Insert chapter ten text here. Insert chapter ten text here. Insert chapter ten text here. Insert chapter ten text here. Insert chapter ten text here. Insert chapter ten text here. Insert chapter ten text here. Insert chapter ten text here. Insert chapter ten text here. Insert chapter ten text here. Insert chapter ten text here. Insert chapter ten text here.

Insert chapter ten text here. Insert chapter ten text here.

Insert chapter ten text here. Insert chapter ten text here. Insert chapter ten text here. Insert chapter ten text here. Insert chapter ten text here. Insert chapter ten text here. Insert chapter ten text here. Insert chapter ten

text here. Insert chapter ten text here.

Insert chapter ten text here. Insert chapter ten text here.

Insert chapter ten text here. Insert chapter ten text here. Insert chapter ten text here. Insert chapter ten text here. Insert chapter ten text here. Insert chapter ten text here. Insert chapter ten text here.

Insert chapter ten text here. Insert chapter ten text here.

Insert chapter ten text here. Insert chapter ten text here. Insert chapter

ten text here. Insert chapter ten text here. Insert chapter ten text here. Insert chapter ten text here. Insert chapter ten text here. Insert chapter ten text here. Insert chapter ten text here. Insert chapter ten text here. Insert chapter ten text here. Insert chapter ten text here. Insert chapter ten text here. Insert chapter ten text here. Insert chapter ten text here. Insert chapter ten text here. Insert chapter ten text here. Insert chapter ten text here.

ABOUT THE AUTHOR

Insert author bio text here. Insert author bio text here